Acknowledgeme

G000090924

First and foremost, I would like to thank my frien̲ ̲.̲p̲.̲.̲.̲ ̲.̲.̲l̲u̲u̲u̲t̲ ̲u̲e̲r̲,̲ ̲w̲u̲o̲ knows how long I would have gone without knowing the cause of my symptoms. Or how much sicker I would have become in the meantime. She saved me from what looked like inevitable disability—from physical, mental, and emotional suffering. In truth, she saved my life!

I would also like to thank everyone who put up with me while I was sick. I don't know why you did it. I was not a nice person at the time. I couldn't have possibly been any fun to be around, but you stuck by me anyway. Even when I was a forgetful, angry jerk, when I double booked and flaked out, when I was a cranky, foggy mess, you stood by my side. Mishelle, Melisa, Sara, Tim, Shelley, Suzy, and Suzie, thank you for having my back even when I was a big asshole.

Mom, thank you for always being there. Thank you for forgiving my temper. Thank you for understanding when I snapped because the pain in my body and the fog in my head was too much to bear.

And my children, thank you for understanding when I was in too much pain to be the mom I wanted to be for you. I did my best, but now I will do better. Thank you for letting me make up for lost time.

Introduction

I almost didn't write this book. I almost abandoned it altogether after the initial try.

When I first sat down to write about my experiences living with an undiagnosed autoimmune disorder, what came out was nothing more than a bitch-fest. Less than six months had passed since I unraveled the mystery of my waning health. Most of my body had healed. The initial relief had worn off. I was no longer grateful that what had tormented me for so long was just celiac and not something worse. I took my renewed health for granted.

I didn't get very far on that first draft, a few pages at most, and I am thankful for that now. The world has enough negativity, I didn't need to add any more to it.

Time went by and I thought about picking the project up here and there but nothing really came to me. My muse never sang.

My original goal was to help others with undiagnosed celiac disease, but the negativity and the lack of gratitude with which I had approached the subject could not possibly have yielded those results. I decided not to write the book. Nothing good could come of it. At least not in the frame of mind I was in. But I couldn't just keep what I had learned to myself either. That would be selfish. There had to be a middle way.

Months went by and circumstances forced me to take a long hard look in the mirror. I didn't like who I had become. I saw the worst in everything and everyone. Not only did I take my renewed health for granted, I had even let a snippet of bitterness creep in. (*It wasn't fair, I wanted cake too!*)

I couldn't continue like that. I needed a change. I needed to start seeing the good in life. I needed gratitude.

I decided that, moving forward, I would be thankful for all the good in my life. I made lists of what I was thankful for and I found that it is quite a lot. When negative thoughts about my dietary restrictions crept in, I reminded myself to be appreciative for the health I have now.

I recalled how sick I had been just a year prior. My entire body ached: my muscles, my joints, the pain went so deep it felt as though it was radiating through my bones. My mouth was riddled with ulcers that made eating a painful chore. I gained twenty pounds because I couldn't move my body, then lost it plus some more because the ulcers interfered with my caloric intake. My blood pressure was through the roof. I couldn't concentrate. I couldn't write anything remotely intelligible. It was like I was walking around in a fog; a terrible, painful, fog.

I compared where I was then to where I am now. My body has recovered more than I thought possible. Most days I don't even have to remember that I ever had debilitating back pain or arthritis. I can chew, eat, and drink through a straw without interference from sores on my tongue, gums, or cheeks. My pulse and blood pressure are normal and I no longer feel as though I am having one long anxiety attack after another. I can think! I can remember stuff, and process information, and what I write makes sense again.

The more gratitude I felt for my healing, the more I began to see the changes that took place in my body as a miracle, not in a religious manner per se, but rather in the sense that my life has been saved.

It hit me. I could still share my story with others who are suffering if I could do it with gratitude. Once I realized that I could do this I knew I was on the right track. The book I wanted to write finally felt RIGHT. I had to write it, I had to! There are too many people out there with this disease who have not been given proper medical care. Their symptoms have been waved off by doctor after doctor or they've been misdiagnosed and left to lead a life of disability when they could otherwise live full and active lives.

How many people who are suffering at the hands of incompetent medical professionals could be living rich, full lives free of pain, anxiety, high blood pressure, etc. etc. if they just eliminated certain foods from their diet? How many people are hurting because they were not lucky enough to have someone in their lives to do their doctor's job for them like I did?

Maybe it is you or someone you love. Maybe your medical provider also tried to treat your symptoms instead of the autoimmune reaction that was causing them. If you're anything like me maybe you have had lower back pain for years with no history of injury to explain why. Or maybe you had an injury but the pain persists despite it being long since healed.

I can't even begin to count the number of people I have talked to who had an injury one, five, ten, even twenty years prior and they're still suffering even though no nerve damage was done. But their doctors treat them as if this is normal, especially with lower back pain. Lower back pain seems to be a given in the medical community. My medical providers certainly didn't bat an eye or wonder why I was in chronic pain in my mid-30s.

And I didn't need to be! By removing one peptide from my diet I was also able to eliminate lower back pain from my life. Years of my life were spent in unnecessary pain. Years of my life were wasted! But they will be worth it if I can help others solve the mystery of what is going on in their body.

If I had not taken my health into my own hands I would have been a gold mine for Big Pharma.

- Chronic back pain
- Arthritis
- High Blood Pressure
- Insomnia
- Anxiety
- Excessive sweating
- Allergies
- Insanely huge ulcers in my mouth
- Ulcers in my nose
- A scabby, flaky scalp
- Alternating, nausea, diarrhea, constipation, and constipated diarrhea

The list goes on and on. Everything that could have been wrong with me, was. And my medical provider was more than willing to whip out her prescription pad to treat my symptoms as if they were the actual disease.

I was lucky. And smart. I refused to believe that, after being relatively healthy my whole life, my body was simply falling apart from countless different diseases and geriatric maladies at the age of 35.

I was also lucky enough to have a very good friend in the health industry who recognized the symptoms I was experiencing as a probable autoimmune disease. I am eternally grateful to this friend who, with a clinical doctorate in physical therapy, often sees what so many general practitioners not only missed, but failed to even consider, let alone rule out.

It wasn't my friend's job to take over where my doctor failed, but she cared and took the time to listen and that made all the difference in the world. I am convinced that this woman saved my life. Simply put, I cannot thank her enough. If it were not for her I would probably be languishing on disability right now, my health and life destroyed by something avoidable.

Which is exactly why I had to write this book, I had to share this miracle with the world. And I must tell my story because I know there are others who will read it, see their own mysterious combination of symptoms, and receive healing accordingly. It is with this attitude of gratitude that I decided to write this book after all, so that I can give back, and hopefully help others find the healing that they so desperately need.

Chapter One

All the Hate

I didn't appreciate my health until after I got super sick and then better again. Even after the muscles in my back and legs felt like they were eating themselves alive, I was not grateful for the strong body I had prior to getting ill. When my hands were in constant pain, my knuckles were stiff, and I dropped things constantly; even then I was not thankful for the time prior when my hands worked perfectly fine and were free and clear of any signs of debilitating arthritis.

The same is true of when my elbows started to burn so bad they would wake me up multiple times per night; and when at least one knee would ache with every step. I didn't appreciate the time before when my elbows and knees worked as they should, in silent acquiescence, without complaint of pain.

When my mouth filled with huge painful ulcers that made me not want to eat, I didn't appreciate not having holes in my mouth until after they had healed.

The list goes on and on just like my symptoms. It's not something I am proud of and it certainly does not reflect well on who I used to be.

Who I used to be. Whether we are conscious of it or not, we all do change. For better or for worse, I am not the same person I was twenty years ago, ten years ago, five years ago, even six months ago. And I am not the same person I will be in the future. We all go through revolutions, some of them good, some of them bad.

The torment of living with an undiagnosed autoimmune disorder for at least a couple of decades changed me for the worse, but it couldn't have done so if I had not let it. The sicker I got, the less gratitude I had, and the more I disliked people. Really disliked them, in an unhealthy way. At one point, I even hated people.

I hated people who walked too slow or drove too slow. I hated people who took up an entire aisle at the grocery store, their cart left at an angle across the aisle oblivious to the fact that no one could get around them.

I hated people who took up too much space, period.

I was working as a bartender, which has its place for disliking certain people, don't get me wrong. But I hated almost everyone. I hated customers who didn't know what they wanted. I hate customers who knew what they wanted because they had heard of it somewhere but had no idea what it was and stared blankly when asked the simple question, 'Do you want that as a shot or as a martini?' I hated customers who ordered labor intensive drinks and didn't tip. They were almost always one and the same and they were almost always overdressed females barely old enough to drink. I really, really hated those girls.

I hated customers who gave me shit for carding them and they were all of 23.

I hated the customers who would stand at the far end of the bar and make me walk to them. I hated them even more because they never seemed to be able to complete all their transactions at one time. First, they would hand me a video lottery ticket to cash, which forced me to walk back to the other end of the bar. My back would stiffen and cramp as I walked, a jolt of pain radiated down my right leg with every step. After I returned with their winnings, on this third trip across the bar, and counted back their money, they would ask to trade in their 20-dollar bills for fives. Even if I tried to preempt this and ask ahead of time if they would need fives, they almost never did. Until I got back with their money and I would have to return to the register a second time.

I really hated those people. I cursed at them in my head along with every painful step.

I would return with their fives, then they would order a beer.

Stupid mutherf . . .

And then they would hand me one of the fives I just gave them. As if they couldn't have paid for their beer with the twenty to begin with, gotten their fives in change, and saved me from hobbling the length of the bar two extra times.

Hope you get runover by a car on your way home!

My inner dialogue was out of control. Like I said, I hated people. I was not in a good spot. Chronic pain had done me in.

Chapter Two

Pain, Pain Go Away

After any given eight-hour bartending shift, I drove home with tears in my eyes. Pain shot down my back, through my right leg, all the way down my calf. When I got home I couldn't even sit on my couch because of the spasms in my back and right leg. I sat on the floor and cried while I ran an Epsom salt bath in hopes of a little relief.

I was 35 and crawling out of bed like an elderly woman because the ache in my joints and muscles was so intense.

Any time I injured myself or over did it and something started to hurt, it never stopped, it became a chronic part of my life.

In February of 2015 I went on holiday in Vancouver, B.C. I went for a long walk my first day there, only to pay the price on and off for over a year. The walk was nothing new, it is an extremely walkable city and I usually traverse downtown multiple times on foot when I visit. The difference at this point was how bad the disease had ravaged my intestines, and how few vitamins and minerals I was absorbing.

The back of my left knee began to ache.

I hadn't done anything to injure it (whatever that would be). I had not hyperextended it or tripped or fallen off a curb. Literally all I had done was walk.

Sometimes the pain eased for a few days, even a few weeks, at a time. But eventually it always came back.

Just prior to that particular trip to B.C. I began an internship at a nano brewery in Portland Oregon. Part of my job was banging the bungs into the old-school kegs (yes that's a real thing!). When I mentioned to the brewer how my elbow hurt from smacking the bung with the sand weighted hammer he thought it was weird. He didn't have any issues, and he banged a lot more bungs than I did. He had been banging bungs for years and years. And he didn't know anyone else in the industry who complained about aching or burning elbows either—it wasn't a thing like tennis elbow.

My elbow continued to hurt even after my internship ended. Then my left elbow, which had never been involved in banging a single bung, started to burn. It felt like it was on fire! Often it caused more pain than the right one.

It didn't make sense, but they both continued to ache and burn for months and months to come.

As an aside, I think I should point out that I am by no means a wuss. I don't cry over papercuts, or refrain from slicing lemons when I have one. Twisting my ankle doesn't even phase me anymore. I gave birth to a beautiful seven-and-a-half-pound girl without any drugs. I find tattoos soothing, not painful. Yesterday I dropped one of those thick gaudy bottles of True Religion — the big 3.5 ounce one — smack dab on a single toe. I haven't let the hematoma that developed stop me from going down the stairs to the pool or walking across the street for a bottle of chocolate milk. (Don't judge me on the chocolate milk okay, I'm not ashamed to admit I love it!)

My point is, I am not exaggerating the level of pain I was in. Every step hurt but it also hurt to stand, sit, or lay down. On the right side of my body my foot, then my lower leg, and finally my hip went numb when I stood too long, which was all the time since I worked on my feet. Sometimes if I sat too long in one position the numbness travelled upwards instead, reaching my face. My hands went numb a lot too. My elbows throbbed and burned. My shoulders ached. I was losing strength and range of motion, especially in the left shoulder. Arthritis racked my joints. Just about every muscle in my body was afflicted with myopathy—weak, broken down, and lumpy to the touch. My body screamed at me as I tried to climb out of bed in the morning. It raged at me over everyday activities. I gave up and crashed out on the couch long before the day was done. Everything I did hurt. Everything. It is because I am not a wuss, because I constantly forced myself to push on despite the agony, and because I was so determined to live up to my responsibilities, that I did not give up and let the pain win.

Chapter Three

Mystery Symptoms

It wasn't just bodily pain that assailed me either. I suffered from a whole host of physical, emotional, and mental symptoms.

My blood pressure was through the roof. Where it had been 120 over 80 my whole life, the year I got really sick the systolic (top) number had climbed to the 160s. I had palpitations all the time, especially when I was trying to sleep. Two beats would come too quick, too close together, or it would miss a beat altogether, then another in the next breath.

My resting heart rate was over 140 beats per minute. It felt as though my heart were going to jump out of my chest at the exact same time that it felt as though it could just stop beating at any moment.

I was freaking out all the time too, in a constant state of anxiety. I worried about everything, so that when I worried about one thing it brought up everything else I could possibly worry about. I couldn't see the forest for the trees.

I forgot everything too: appointments, deadlines, paying the bills before the lights got shut off.

My brain was in a fog. I couldn't think straight. Whenever I tried to plot a novel or other writing project my head felt thick, my thoughts slow and viscous. When I tried to write, I would get stuck. Stuck mid-sentence, mid-paragraph, mid-chapter.

Where I had written numerous fictional novels in the years leading up to this, the year I got really, really sick I tried to write the last book in my middle grade sci-fi trilogy Left Behind, and failed miserably. It was absolute rubbish. Now that I have my faculties back to normal I have my work cut out for me in the rewrite department. And after rereading it, I am a little embarrassed that I ever sent it out to beta readers in the first place. My brain was such sludge that I didn't even recognize how bad it was at the time. I probably owe each of them an apology.

This wasn't just writer's block either. It got to the point where I could not even articulate concrete thoughts to other people without losing my train of thought in the process.

My head hurt constantly. It was one of those dull aches that is easy to get used to but is also very draining at the same time. I couldn't really take anything for it. Like the back pain, I had to learn to deal with the headaches. There are only so many anti-inflammatories a person can swallow before they start to worry about their liver and kidneys and other vital organs. Besides, ibuprofen made my ankles swell even more.

My ankles were always swollen too. For as long as I can remember, I was a skinny girl with cankles. Yes, even at 120 pounds, I had dimples on the insides of my ankles.

I developed scabs on my scalp. Like dandruff on steroids.

At my worst, I often couldn't eat. When I did, my mouth ached and stung. Ulcers over a centimeter across developed under and along the sides of my tongue, on the insides of my cheeks, and sometimes even at the gum line. Clusters of smaller ulcers appeared, ten or more grouped together. They weren't as deep so they weren't as bad, but they still hurt for as long as they were present, they still turned meals into pure torture. Those ones were usually flat and white, whereas the bigger ones were definite holes, often a millimeter deep. At any given time, I had upwards of thirty ulcers in my mouth between the gaping holes and the groups of smaller sores. My frenulum would scab over with little white patches. Just moving my tongue to drink through a straw made it ache. I also suffered from dry mouth and the salivary glands under my tongue were swollen and hard.

Nothing ever tasted quite right either. I loved food, but I could no longer enjoy it. Ironically this was also the heaviest point in my life, excluding pregnancies. I couldn't exercise anymore. My previous athletic prowess was gone, my physical abilities were drained, it took everything I had just to go to work. And even that felt like it was killing me.

I hit 148.

Okay, okay, I can hear the snickers. *148, that ain't shit!* I get it. A lot of people would be over the moon to weigh under 150 pounds. But on my small frame? I felt like I was suffocating.

Even if it weren't for the pain, I wouldn't have been able to run (my favorite form of exercise) at that weight. I was out of breath just going up a flight of stairs. And I was just plain uncomfortable being that heavy, no matter how good the curves looked on me. My clothes didn't fit and it sapped my energy, which I had less and less of as I avoided eating with the ulcers in my mouth. I was fat and hungry, what a combination! Eventually I started to drop weight. A lot of it, and quick.

It wasn't just my tongue and mucus membranes that suffered either, my teeth did too. Except for breaking one of my front teeth in half when I was a silly, daredevil kid, I never needed any dental work. The one occasion a dentist claimed I had cavities, time and a second opinion proved him wrong. Then, out of nowhere, the enamel started to wear away at my gum line.

It was a slow process, so slow that I didn't really notice what was happening until one day I looked at my gum line and wondered where the enamel had gone. Something had done significant damage to my teeth, but I hadn't changed anything in my diet or lifestyle that could account for it. Like the rest of my health problems, it was a mystery.

Anger settled in. Where I had always been a bit high strung, I became angry constantly. Really angry. And I never took a break from it. Of course, being anxious and foggy and forgetful only made it worse. Or maybe those symptoms caused it . . . chicken . . . egg . . . that whole thing . . . who knows). Of course, being in a constant state of rage made me not a very nice person.

Like most people, I took it out on the ones I love. That was probably the worst symptom of all, and it is the one I have to watch out for even now that the rest of my body has mostly healed. I allowed anger to become a habit, a way of life. So even though I do not have anywhere near the rage I had before, I am still prone to a temper that flares.

I cannot possibly overemphasize how little energy I had when I was ill. It got so bad that I was in bed over twelve hours a day on most days. I did not sleep twelve hours a day, but I spent that much time there just trying to sleep. Most of the time I couldn't sleep. When I could, it never seemed to be effective. I never woke up energized. I never wanted to get out of bed.

I was so, so, so very tired.

I had dealt with insomnia my whole life, but this was beyond insomnia. Even when I slept, I had nothing. I was zapped, depleted, barely making it through the average work day.

Where I had always prided myself on the home cooked meals I prepared for my two beautiful children, I began to rely on fast food more and more. Five-dollar Little Caesar's pizzas, Jack in the Box, even McDonalds. I was so desperate for food, which I didn't have the strength or energy to prepare, that I turned to rely on the very type of sustenance that should never have been a regular part of my diet. (Or really, anyone's, but especially mine.) And, of course, the more fast food I ate, the sicker I got. It was a horrible treadmill, worse than I could even imagine at the time.

Chapter Four

Tummy Trouble

Then there was my stomach. But it was the last thing on my mind. Intestinal issues had always been a part of my life.

At the time, it wasn't something that I connected to what was happening to the rest of my body because I had been suffering since I was a teenager, whereas the rest of my symptoms did not develop until much, much later. The older I got, the worse my stomach problems became, but it happened so slowly that I did not notice how much worse they were at the time. All I knew was that my digestive system was in turmoil: solid stool was rare and when it did happen it floated at the top of the bowl (as did every type of bowel movement). The bloating I experienced after eating became unbearable, and then there was the constipated diarrhea.

Yes, that is correct, constipated diarrhea. Sounds impossible, right? Well it's not. It is a very real and fucked up thing to have! Thankfully it wasn't constant, it came and went, but when it came it was the most miserable gut situation I could imagine.

All I knew was, I had to poop but I couldn't. I tried colon cleanses. I tried flooding my colon with sodium from extra, extra dirty martinis, then with baking soda dissolved in water. Finally, I tried eating extra spicy food. Bad idea. Not only did the heat not work, but when I finally was able to go, oh boy did it burn! I don't want to get too graphic here, but it was like trying to push hot lava out of my butt.

Furthermore, I was always nauseous. I never got a break from it. I smoked marijuana multiple times a day for relief. It got to the point where I couldn't even eat without smoking weed first.

Not only did I have zero appetite, but even if I was starving, just trying to eat would make me gag as often as not. I would literally put a bite of food in my mouth, attempt to chew, and gag. I would try to swallow it and gag. It was like my body was rejecting food, and as I found out later, with good reason.

Whereas most people gain weight on vacation, I would come back from a three-day holiday at least five pounds lighter. I was over the moon when medical dispensaries became a thing anyone with ten minutes to see a doctor (for free!) could access in British Columbia. I no longer had to decide between eating and smuggling marijuana across the border (which I was too scared to do anyway).

So, I was medicating to eat and I was also medicating to fall asleep. And then again to go back to sleep.

I took the insomnia as a given too. Going to sleep was a battle ever since I was a teenager and it got worse each year. In fact, it got to the point where I would lay there for hours and hours only to fall asleep for a fraction as long and then start the process all over again. A lot of people go through this and can confirm, it is pure torture.

When I discovered that smoking a little herb would help put me out back in college, I felt like I had found a miracle cure. But the sicker I got, the more I had to smoke to sleep. The same was true with my appetite. If I wanted to eat I had to smoke more weed than ever before. And sometimes even that didn't work.

It wasn't tolerance. The anti-"drug" people are wrong. It didn't take any more to get me high, that never changed. It was that so much damage had been done to my body and my psyche that I was losing my ability to function, and marijuana was no longer enough to get me by.

I needed a true miracle. I needed healing.

Chapter Five

Doctor, Doctor

Going to the doctor is not exactly my idea of a good time. I go once a year like every healthy lady should (stop putting these off, they can save your life!) but other than that I try to avoid it. Most things get better on their own with time anyway, like that toe I nearly crushed with a bottle of perfume. So why waste an afternoon waiting to see a Nurse Practitioner who is just going to tell me to ice it and avoid reinjuring it? Unless I feel like I'm dying, I generally avoid going into the clinic.

When I got really, really, really sick, I felt like I was dying. I went to the doctor four times that year.

Work was tearing my back up. Twisting, pivoting, sliding and pulling cooler doors open, these are all things that bartenders do throughout the course of a shift without a second thought. Until they hurt. Every. Single. Time.

Walking. Bending. Stooping.

My back was stiff as a board but I could still touch my toes.

The pain had started years before. It started out mild and the buildup was slow but it got steadily worse, so that I didn't notice how bad it was or how much it was affecting my life until one day I realized that not only did it hurt more often than it didn't, but that tipping point had long since passed. In fact, there was never a time when it didn't hurt any more.

I couldn't remember the last time my back was pain free.

My life had been severely hampered but I had only just begun noticing to what degree. I have always adjusted to the difficulties in my life and gone on, pain was no different. But my life was affected in ways that I wish I could go back in time and un-do.

I couldn't teach my daughter to ride a two-wheeler. I couldn't run alongside of her or support the bike or catch her if she started to fall.

I couldn't run at all.

I was no longer much help to friends who needed assistance hauling furniture and boxes up and down a flight of stairs or two. I tried. I gave it my best when one of my closest friends needed help moving apartments. I kept going even though the lightest loads wrenched my back. The stairs alone made it seize and spasm. I bowed out on the heavy furniture though. At least

I was smart enough not to let pride lay me out for the next day or two.

It wasn't right. There was no way I was supposed to be in this much pain. And from what? I had never had an injury. And it certainly wasn't old age. I called in for an appointment.

My assigned provider was not available so I saw the on-call practitioner instead. She asked me why I was there but she did not pose any follow up questions.

Her: What are you here for today?

Me: Lower back pain. It's affecting my job. I have to work.

Her: What kind of pain is it? Stabbing? Shooting? Burning? Aching?

Me: All of them.

Her: (writes script) Here, this might make you drowsy, but it should help.

She didn't examine me. She didn't ask what made it worse or if anything made it feel better. She didn't ask me if I had ever been injured.

If she had bothered to ask about how and when my back first began to hurt I would have had to tell her an embarrassing story about how, when it came time for a new mattress, I made the mistake of purchasing a pillowtop where a firm mattress would have better suited my tummy sleeping habits. I would have had to admit that I sat on this mattress while I wrote a tragic comedy about a guy who hires a hitman to off himself even though it hurt my back the entire time. And I would have to admit that I had worn five-inch heels on more than one occasion.

If she had bothered to ask maybe she would have realized that the pain I was experiencing was out of line with the only causes I could come up with. Maybe she would have realized that there had to be an underlying problem. Probably not, since she gave me a prescription for Vicodin and sent on my way without so much as a manual exam of my lower back.

Vicodin? Seriously? I was on my feet for eight to ten hours at a time. I needed relief. I needed to work without being in pain every time I had to reach or stoop for something. I didn't need to be high on an opiate.

I started seeing a chiropractor, which I paid out of pocket for. It did wonders at first but I could also think of a ton of other things I could spend that $55 a pop on (or *pop, pop, pop, pop, pop*).

I knew I wasn't supposed to be in so much pain. Something needed to be done. A month or so later I called for another appointment. I did not want to, but I had to go back. This time my assigned provider was available.

It was the first time I had ever met her. Like I said, I don't go in for every sneeze or sniffle. My previous provider had retired since the last time I was in. This one immediately flicked me shit. She assumed I was drug seeking and told me straight out she wouldn't give me any more Vicodin.

As if it were my fault her incompetent crony had written the Rx in the first place!

I was insulted. I was hardly after drugs! What I was after, what I hoped for, was physical therapy.

Not covered.

What about my chiropractor?

Not covered.

"But you should get a massage instead," she said.

To her credit, she did order x-rays and she did at least examine me. "The muscles in your back are very tight." Well duh. "But you have excellent range of motion."

I could still touch my toes. I could still stretch. Stretching was about all I could do at the time.

She admonished me to get more exercise without ever asking me about my routine or lack thereof (and this from a woman more than twice as big around as me). I was close to tears. I loved exercising! I loved to run! My back didn't hurt because I stopped running, I stopped running because I couldn't stand the pain anymore.

Like her co-worker, she didn't bother to ask me about when or how my back had started to hurt, or even if I had ever had a specific injury. Maybe I am being silly, but I would think those would be some of the first questions any provider would ask when a patient presents with chronic pain.

She sent me to a pain clinic.

A pain clinic? I had no idea what that was but she made it sound like they would help me rehab my aching back. That wasn't at all what they were in the business of, but she let me believe it as she handed me a prescription for muscle relaxers, another for an anti-inflammatory, a sheet of paper with diagrams of stretches that were supposed to loosen up my back, and told me that the pain clinic would call me.

That was twice in about a month's time that I went into see my medical provider over back pain. I wasn't even at the worst of it yet. That wouldn't come for at least six more months. Did I bother going back then? Of course not. They weren't going to help me. The pain clinic my provider sent me to was a joke. It wasn't designed to help me heal or get better. It was designed to give me the skills to live with chronic pain for the rest of my life.

Seriously. Those were the clinician's words at orientation.

My heart sunk. Was I really going to deal with this for the rest of my life? It didn't seem right.

Meanwhile, while my back got worse, I started getting rashes of what I thought were canker sores in my mouth. They were just small white lesions that hurt whenever I ate or drank anything acidic or if my teeth grazed against them.

I didn't think much of them at first. They came and went with no seeming rhyme or reason. Then they got bigger—and that's when then they became actual holes. And they were everywhere inside of my mouth: inside my cheeks, on my gums, on the sides of my tongue as well as under it. They were on the inside of my lips and sometimes they would peek out so that I worried people would think I was diseased.

The salivary glands underneath my tongue swelled up and got hard. My mouth was as dry as a desert. No amount of water could moisten it. Sometimes I would take a drink and just hold the water in my mouth for some relief. Scabby white patches covered my frenulum and it hurt to even move my tongue.

By the early winter of 2016 I couldn't take it anymore. The sores in my mouth were so bad that I could barely eat. I called for an appointment. Once again, my regular doctor wasn't available. Once again, I saw the on-call provider.

She took one look and told me it was herpes.

It wasn't. I knew it wasn't. I was flabbergasted. I didn't know what to say, other than to argue, "I don't have herpes." Lame, I know.

She ordered a blood test and then cancelled it after I told her that she could go through my records and see that I get tested at least every year for all things sexually transmissible. She still sent in a script for herpes medication and some sort of oral rinse that was supposed to help alleviate the pain.

When I went to the pharmacy to pick up the rinse the pharmacist didn't understand the instructions so it wasn't ready. But they had that damn herpes medication all packaged and labeled and ready to go. I refused it. I am not an idiot and I was not going to take a medication for something I knew I didn't have.

Chapter Six

Someone to Listen

The evening after that entirely useless trip to the clinic, I almost didn't keep plans to meet a friend at a local tap house for a few beers. I felt like crap. My mouth ached. My stomach ached. My whole body ached. At that point in my life it was kind of dumb of me to even make plans in the first place. I ALWAYS considered cancelling them. But I made it to the tap house and I even found a parking spot that wasn't too far away, something I never cared about until every step stabbed at my lower back and sent a jolt of pain down my right leg.

I don't know why this friend wanted to spend any kind of time with me. The last time I had seen her I was in a foul mood and today wasn't any different. Chronic pain had taken its toll and I didn't have anything nice to say about anything, but at least I peppered my negativity with a hearty self-deprecating laugh, so I guess there's that.

Sometimes all you can do is joke about your own misfortune, right?

I joked, but I did a lot of complaining too. I complained about the sores in my mouth and how every sip of beer I took hurt, every bite of chips and salsa felt like acid and rocks in my mouth. I complained about how hungry I was. And how fat I felt.

I complained about the doctor I had gone to see earlier that day.

"It's not herpes," I told her. "I know it's not."

My friend, who happens to be a physical therapist with a clinical doctorate, looked at me kind of strange and asked if I had joint pain too.

Did I have joint pain? DID I HAVE JOINT PAIN?!

How did she know? I hadn't mentioned anything about my elbows that burned so badly they woke me up throughout the night. Or my aching knees, the right one that hurt at the kneecap and the left one that hurt in the crook. Nor had I said a thing about my stiff hands and fingers or how those small joints cracked and ached.

She asked if I had ever heard of Bechet's. When she saw the look on my face, she took it back quick. She told me not to worry about it, I wasn't in a wheelchair, it was a rare disease. She described a client who she worked with. They had the same sores I did and their joint pain was such that they depended on a wheelchair to get around. I was way, way, way better off than this person was.

It might have been a flip statement, but she saved my life that night by putting two and two together. Something auto-immune was going on.

Chapter Seven

Missed Diagnosis

Something auto-immune had been going on for a very long time. Since at least high school I had experienced a strange litany of seemingly disconnected symptoms that were mild enough to ignore once I visited my medical provider and received a prompt misdiagnosis.

The first time I went to the doctor for stomach trouble was in either my sophomore or junior year of high school. My stomach hurt constantly. I missed at least one day a week of school because of the cramps and bloating and diarrhea that assailed me. For some reason, my mom thought I might have an ulcer and made me an appointment with the doctor.

Perhaps I should note here that most of the medical professionals I have seen over the years have been Nurse Practitioners, not Medical Doctors. This is common practice in managed healthcare, and yet in our culture we say, "I am going to the doctor." Even though chances are the person we are seeing is not technically an MD, no one says, "I don't feel well, I think I will go see my nurse practitioner." In keeping with the popular vernacular, I do refer to medical providers who (mis)treated me as doctors if I do not recall their technical status.

I don't know if this particular provider was a Medical Doctor or a Nurse Practitioner, but she began with questions about my life: home, school, the works. Before examining me, she determined that I must be under a lot of stress.

The exam itself was brief. She pressed on various parts of my stomach and determined that, no, I did not have an ulcer. She did not give me a blood test for H. Pylori, the bacteria that is the major cause of peptic ulcers, or run any blood tests for that matter.

She did not consider any other possible causes or diseases. She did not rule out a more serious illness like stomach cancer or autoimmune disorders like Crohn's or celiac before she decided that what was ailing me was simply that I was freaking the fuck out.

"Stress." That was her diagnosis and I accepted it.

I mean, I was under a lot of stress at the time. My family life wasn't exactly perfect. My younger brother was struggling and the rest of us were reacting. My parents were divorced and not on amicable terms. It was nothing worse than what anyone else I knew was going through, but still, it WAS stressful.

Obviously neither my mom or I were medical doctors, so we accepted the diagnosis and I went on with life without any kind of treatment. Seriously. If stress were my issue, why wasn't I given meditation techniques at the very least? Or even a stress ball?

Facetiousness aside, I went on suffering with the admonition of "Try to be less stressed out." Yeah, sure, as a fifteen or sixteen-year-old kid I definitely had the tools to do that, right?

It would not have mattered if I did. Stress was never the issue. True, it may have exacerbated my tummy trouble, but it was never the cause.

I didn't go back to the doctor for those relentless stomach problems until I was 30. And that wasn't because I didn't need to—I hadn't gotten any better. I suffered the entire while. Every time I ate, my stomach would bloat up. If I went to a buffet or ate too much, my stomach would cramp and I would be forced to rush to the toilet. I had diarrhea constantly. It was like a way of life.

Somewhere in my mid-twenties nausea joined the rest of the symptoms that assaulted my stomach and I just went with it. After all, everyone knows stress can do a number on your tummy, right?

But by 30 I couldn't take it anymore. My tummy trouble had become acute and unbearable. For weeks, I was so nauseous that I was actually throwing up. My stomach burned. My bowel movements burned (even without spicy foods). I tried colon cleanses. I tried swearing off soda (especially Coca Cola) and dairy. When I couldn't make it to work because I was stuck on the toilet, I knew I needed to see someone. I dreaded what I already knew they would say.

And yes, I was under a tremendous amount of stress at the time. In addition to being a single mom to a toddler and a tween, my job was becoming increasingly difficult, as I had taken a promotion that basically required me to sign off on other people's fraudulent lies. Meanwhile the agency I worked for was experiencing funding cuts, which meant more work and less pay for everyone. So, when the doctor said, "It's probably stress," I bought it.

Surprisingly, he did order a battery of blood tests and an ultrasound just to make sure there wasn't anything else going on. But while he checked my liver and kidney function and tested for cancer, he did not mention any need to test for celiac, or order a biopsy of my intestines to check the status of my villi. He never mentioned Chron's or that I should try an elimination, gluten free, or FODMAP diet.

Looking back, my mind is still boggled by this. How can a patient report fifteen years of persistent, worsening gut trouble and neither celiac or Chron's be considered?

The tests showed nothing. Of course, they were the wrong tests. Once again, I was told stress was the culprit and sent on my way. And once again, I bought it and went on suffering.

I returned to that same doctor a few months later when I developed an ulcer in my nose. I was working as a case manager for disability services in the Medicaid program at the time and I regularly met clients in their homes and hospital rooms, right along with their contagious diseases. MRSA was one of those and I was a little freaked out that the ulcer could be from the relentless staph bug. How many clients had I had who went from having a little sore to being hospitalized for a blood infection?

Plenty. The answer is plenty.

Thank goodness it wasn't MRSA. I was young and healthy and I really didn't have anything to worry about. But that doesn't mean I got the proper diagnosis either.

The doctor did a visual inspection of my affected nostril and wrote me a prescription for Allegra. Yes, that is correct, he put me on allergy medication.

I left his office befuddled, though he wasn't entirely wrong. While the allergy medication didn't do anything for the ulcer, that one went away and came back off and on, it did improve my breathing and cleared my sinuses. So, I had developed allergies, he was right about that, but the ulcer wasn't part of them. And, in fact, even my allergies went away when I discovered what was actually wrong with me.

It was around this time that I started developing lower back pain, but I wasn't about to go back to the doctor. I chalked it up to bad posture while I wrote Suicide in Tiny Increments from my overly soft bed and the ridiculous heels I wore to work and out on the weekends. I told myself it was my fault, that it would get better when I bought a new mattress and wrote from a desk like a normal person. I didn't bother seeing a doctor for my back until years later, after it got much, much worse. (Chapter Five shows just how well that went.)

There was one other time I went to the doctor for a random symptom that turned out to be caused by the same undiagnosed auto-immune disorder. I was in my mid-twenties and this time it was for something even more embarrassing than ongoing diarrhea: excessive sweating.

I was constantly sweating through my clothes and I was sick of it. The problem had started years earlier, also in high school, but I found ways to hide it. At first, I wore layers so that the sweat wouldn't show through right away, though it inevitably seeped through each and every one. Next, I turned to wearing a jacket whenever I was in public. Even in the summer. When people thought that was weird, I switched to wearing nothing but black to hide the stains. My fashion choices were severely hampered by the buckets of sweat that poured from my armpits. When I did buy cute non-black tops, they would be stained and ruined after only a few wears.

But I didn't go to the doctor for it until the uniform at a new job forced me to. I couldn't hide my problem anymore, I needed help.

This time the doctor (who was not the same one I saw for my stomach a decade earlier) sent me in for a blood test, but this wasn't the right one either. She thought my overly active sweat glands might be the result of an over active thyroid. It wasn't. She told me that Botox might help, but my insurance wouldn't cover it. What I had to figure out on my own was that it was actually anxiety that was making me perspire. As I paid attention to when I would sweat I noticed that it didn't happen when I was home alone. Or with close family or friends. It happened in social situations where I was anxious. I was already stressed, according to the doctor I had seen for my stomach ten-ish years prior, so I accepted my self-diagnosis and continued to mask my excessive perspiration any way I could, even at work. Little did I know, anxiety was just another one of those mysterious non-intestinal symptoms of the auto-immune disorder that afflicts my body. Nor did I realize just how anxious I was until a decade later when, all of a sudden, a change in my diet made all of my symptoms go away, including ones like this that I didn't even realize were symptoms.

Chapter Eight

Bechet's?

I looked up Bechet's as soon as I arrived home from that fateful meeting at the tap house. My friend told me not to but I did anyway. She knew I would, she even said so much, something to the effect of *you don't have it so don't let what you see freak you out.*

That was certainly easier said than done!

A vascular autoimmune disease . . . affects the eyes, mouth, genitals, joints, and skin . . . I clicked on images. The ulcers looked just like the ones in my mouth. Clusters of small white canker-like sores. Big gaping gashes. Any number of those photographs could have been taken from my mouth at one point or another

There were images of those same sores on genitals. Male and female, both with ulcers right on their most private of private parts. I gasped. My heart raced and I broke out in a cold sweat. I feared such sores were in my future. I was already chronically single, what chance would I have of ever meeting anyone decent if my vagina was rendered unusable by giant ulcers?

And if I thought eating with those things in my mouth hurt . . . whooh . . . I don't even want to think of what it would be like to do anything, ANYTHING, even sit or walk or stand, with an ouchie like that on my vajayjay.

Then there were the eyes. My word, the eyes! They were straight out of a zombie movie. My stomach sank, I felt ill. How could such a terrible disease even exist?

I stared at my own eyes in the mirror. I stared at the pingueculas that had formed, one each on the white inside corners of my eyes, either from too much sun, too much wind, or both. What if they were just the beginning? What if, with time, they grew and expanded over my irises?

My beautiful green eyes. I mourned losing them though they were just as bright and clear as ever. I feared going blind like the people in the photographs, though I still saw just fine so long as I had my glasses. I already had the joint pain and the mouth ulcers, after all. I was convinced the rest was not far behind.

The next day at work was torture. I hobbled around in pain as usual, but this time I had an extra burden to drag around with my aching muscles: my thoughts.

Bechet's.

The name kept bouncing around in my head. Whenever I tweaked my back a little more than usual, or ran my tongue along one of the ulcers in my mouth, it rang out loud and clear.

Bechet's

There is a skin test for the disease but according to the internet there are very few medical providers trained to give and interpret it. The fact that I could write words in my skin with a cocktail straw (Dermatographic urticaria, also known as skin writing disease) had me convinced it was a real possibility the test would be positive, IF I were even able to find a provider to administer it.

I was freaking out!

Bechet's. Bechet's.

It chimed over and over in my head.

BECHET'S!

Chapter Nine

A Host of Auto-Immunities

I got home from work and looked up other autoimmune disorders that could put holes in my mouth. With all of my being, I hoped that whatever was afflicting me, it would be something else, something less intense than Bechet's. My friend also mentioned psoriatic arthritis, so there was that . . . and plenty more. Plus, they all had their own set of accompanying symptoms, many of which I was experiencing without even realizing they were symptoms in the first place. When I looked closely at my body and all the strange ways it was failing me, my eyes were opened to just how many different things had gone wrong with me, though I still managed to get by. Until that point, I just accepted my aches and pains and array of seemingly disconnected symptoms as part of life. I thought my cankles and weak fingernails were just quirks of my DNA. I never thought it could all be part of a larger disease process.

I had symptoms spread across a whole host of autoimmune diseases. It could have been anything, I realized as I continued searching the internet for possibilities, it could even be more than one disease. As many medical sites pointed out, often people with one autoimmune disease go on to develop others.

There was Rheumatoid Arthritis, with its joint pain, fatigue, dry mouth, and oral sores that also looked just like the painful holes that developed in my mouth. My mom had recently been diagnosed with R.A. but she is twice my age.

There was Lupus, which also causes joint pain, chronic fatigue, and ulcers in the mouth. In addition, it can cause many of the other symptoms I was experiencing: dry eyes, shortness of breath, headaches, memory problems, and general confusion.

Crohn's could explain my constant digestive problems and floating stools, as well as the sores in my mouth, the constant fatigue I was experiencing, and the pain in my joints.

Sjogren's Syndrome could account for my chronically dry eyes and mouth, swollen salivary glands, fatigue, and aching joints. Since it oftentimes accompanies R.A. and Lupus, it was completely possible that I could have Sjogren's working in tandem with another autoimmune disease to produce the multitude of symptoms I was experiencing.

Psoriatic Arthritis could cause my joint pain, oral ulcers, and the scaly patches of itchy, flaking skin on my scalp.

The next day, I went back to work in a daze. The diseases pinged through my mind one by one. Bechet's. Crohn's. Rheumatoid Arthritis. Lupus. Sjogren's. Psoriasis.

They were all terrible. I cried at the thought of having any of them. Why me? What had I done wrong? I had been fit and healthy until suddenly my body gave up on me. I had taken good care of it, exercised, and eaten more vegetables than average, for this? For an autoimmune disease to ravage my body and steal my life from me?

It was a cycle that went on for days. I went home from work and read more online. I compared my symptoms to disease after disease. Then I went to work the next day and let my thoughts stew, only to come home and read more, look for more clues. Yes, I was driving myself crazy, but how else was I supposed to put together the puzzle? How else was I supposed to solve the mystery? How else was I supposed to get better?

Chapter Ten

Enter the AIP

There were six televisions in the bar I worked at. It seemed like a moment did not go by that there wasn't an advertisement for Humira playing on at least one of them. It was like when you get your period for the first time and you just can't stop noticing the commercials for pads and tampons and such. Humira was everywhere.

Humira for this! Humira for that! Humira for everything!

Humira is an anti-inflammatory that is used to treat different autoimmune disorders, including R.A. and psoriatic arthritis. It was taunting me. It seemed to be saying, "This is your future!" At the end, where they list the medication's side effects, my knees would go weak.

This couldn't be my life. I wouldn't let it be my life.

All these autoimmune diseases, with their ulcers and joint pain, they were all terrible. And so were their treatments. I refused to live a life on anti-inflammatories and pain pills.

I turned back to the internet and stumbled upon the Paleo Auto Immune Protocol (AIP) diet. Its proponents claimed that by eliminating inflammatory foods and healing leaky gut, people with autoimmune diseases could drastically improve their quality of life. Many were even able to go off their medications.

From what I had heard about the Paleo diet, I was skeptical at first. I was under the mistaken impression that Paleo meant massive amounts of animal protein and not much else. But at that point I was willing to try anything that would make me better without making me worse, so I kept reading anyway and decided to give it a go.

The purpose of the Paleo AIP diet is to eliminate all potentially inflammatory foods and foods that can irritate intestinal lining and replace them with nutrient dense foods for at least 30 days (though 90 is often suggested) to allow the leaky gut to heal. It was a long list:

- No dairy
- No eggs.
- No grains (or products made from grains such as malt vinegar or soy sauce).
- No soy.
- No corn.
- No nuts or seeds.

- No beans or legumes.
- No nightshades (tomatoes, eggplant, potatoes, bell peppers, hot peppers, etc.)
- No nitrites or sulfates.
- No alcohol.
- No soda or lemonade or the like.
- No coffee.
- No protein shakes.
- No grapeseed, canola, corn or other vegetable cooking/salad oils.
- No added sugar or sugar substitutes
- Most spices were off limits (paprika comes from a nightshade, for example).
- No processed foods.

The foods I could eat were nutrient dense, meant to heal leaky gut, and the list was much shorter:

- Meat & seafood/fish (preferably high-quality grass-fed meat, no processed meats with nitrites or sulfates, and limited chicken due to high Omega 6 content).
- Offal.
- Vegetables (except nightshades).
- Fruit (except nightshades), limit to two servings a day due to sucrose content.
- Herbs.
- Extra virgin olive oil for dressings, coconut oil for cooking.
- Vinegar (but not malt vinegar).
- Bone broth.
- Kombucha

There are a few different variations on the Paleo AIP diet. Some are less strict and allow different oils as well as nuts. I decided to go with the strictest version I could find (https://www.thepaleomom.com/start-here/the-autoimmune-protocol/) Might as well go big or not at all, right?!

The hardest part of the diet was that, despite my misconceptions of what paleo was, this was not supposed to be a low carbohydrate diet. Somehow, I was supposed to eat carbs with every meal. But how does one eat carbs at every meal without rice, wheat, rye, barley, couscous, oatmeal, or corn? I racked my brain for a carbohydrate that wasn't a grain. I couldn't think of anything.

I read through the diet again. I would have to rely on starchy vegetables.

I perked up a bit. Like potatoes?

Nope, not like potatoes. Those are nightshades. But sweet potatoes were fine, so were their friends the yams. Beets, were an option. As were parsnips. I didn't know how to prepare either but a google search assured me that beets could be delicious boiled.

They weren't.

Plantains were on the list. If you are what you eat, I became a plantain during the 60 days I followed AIP.

The tree vegetable that looks like an oversized banana is very versatile. When it is green and starchy it cooks up like a potato. When it is bright yellow with black streaks, basically when it looks like a rotten banana, then it is sweet like fruit. Fruit that must be cooked, but sweet nonetheless. I preferred them that way and ate plantains almost every day for three months. I also ate a lot of sweet potato during that time. A lot! I don't think I need to share anymore about my bowel movements, but you can imagine what color it was on a diet with a serving of sweet potatoes at most meals.

Chapter Eleven

A Quick Change

It was a very healthy diet, rich in nutrients. And it was a lot of work. Quick meals were a thing of the past. Everything I ate had to be prepared from scratch and cooked. It was intense. And it was a constant puzzle to try and figure out combinations of foods were simultaneously allowed on the diet, tasted good together, and filled me up. It took a while to find a groove, to figure out what to buy at the store, and what to prepare together. At first, I went hungry a lot, but eventually I figured it out.

Breakfast had always been so easy. A bowl of Chex with a sliced-up banana. Oatmeal with brown sugar, milk, and raisins. Plain yogurt with berries, walnuts, and sesame seeds. Bacon, eggs, and toast. Not anymore.

None of my go to foods would work. I couldn't have cereal, cold or hot. I couldn't have brown sugar or milk or yogurt or walnuts or sesame seeds. Or eggs or toast. I could have the bacon if it was nitrite and nitrate free but it probably wasn't. I could have the banana and the berries, but then I wouldn't be allowed to have any more fruit for the rest of the day.

(Confession—I almost always went over the allotted servings of fruit.)

Breakfast did not look like breakfast anymore on the Paleo AIP diet. Typically, I ended up with a ripe plantain sautéed in coconut oil, or a roasted sweet potato with garlic cloves and a little salt. (A small amount of pink Himalayan salt was okay because of the trace minerals, but pepper could irritate the stomach lining so it was out. So much for conventional ideas of 'healthy'.) The starchy carb was then accompanied by a salad of arugula, berries, and olive oil. Yes. A salad. At breakfast. So, what? There was usually a can of sardines involved as well. Sometimes I ate some olives or an avocado too, depending on how hungry I was.

Lunch was a variation of the same thing. If I had plantain in the morning, then I made sweet potato in the afternoon, and vice versa. There would be more arugula for lunch, or spinach maybe, with more olive oil, maybe a little balsamic vinegar, cucumber, and red onions to top it off. Or a roasted vegetable: cauliflower, broccoli, zucchini, asparagus, they all crisped up well with a little garlic. There was always some sort of meat, whether it was another can of sardines or a cut of sirloin off a grass-fed cow. Shrimp, ahi, salmon, tuna, I tried to eat fish or seafood every day in addition to the sardines. It was spendy, but I was determined to get better, to heal my body. And I believed in the power of food to do so.

For dinner, I made things like oxtail soup and roasts that would provide leftovers for a couple of days to come. And I roasted more vegetables, made another salad.

I took fermented cod liver oil at night and drank a mason jar of bone broth at least a couple of times per day. There was always a crockpot full of onion, carrot, garlic cloves, chicken feet, and some kind of bones going — a constant supply of the energy-giving broth. The bones were leftovers from previous meals. Whenever my family had ribs or roasts or chops or any kind of meat with the bone in, I saved that bone for broth. The best broth included bones from more than one kind of animal: beef and pork, pork and chicken, chicken and lamb, lamb and turkey, or beef and pork and chicken, and so on. The best broth had the biggest variety of bones. The worst was when I only had chicken or turkey bones. It's all a matter of taste. Some people like their bone broth with herbs and such, but I stuck with just salt most of the time.

I took vitamins in powder form that were free of additives and cost an arm and a leg. They didn't absorb well in water so I had to cheat a little and use fruit juice (which is discouraged due to sugars). But I went with the lowest sugar and highest fiber content I could find, so don't get too excited. I mixed my vitamins with fucking prune juice, yippee!

I expected it to take at least a couple of weeks before I saw any potential results. It didn't. In a matter of just a couple of days it was obvious that the diet was working—no exaggeration. Right away, the holes in my mouth started to close and heal up. My salivary glands were working again and my dry mouth moistened. Before long I could eat like a normal person. It no longer hurt to chew or simply put food in my mouth. I didn't dread mealtimes any more.

The muscles in my back and legs loosened up immediately. It still hurt to walk, but after only a few days on the AIP diet the pain had lessened enough to be noticeable. The spasms became less and less intense too. I no longer came home from work and sat on the living room floor crying while I waited for my Epsom salt bath. My hips loosened up. In fact, the stiffness and burning in the rest of my joints started to subside as well. I even felt a little less anxious. And the best part? The fog in my brain began to lift.

No, wait, there was one thing better than all those little improvements—I got hope back. The future no longer looked impossible. I knew the day would come when it wouldn't hurt to walk anymore. I saw a future where I could take as many steps as I needed and each one would no longer ache. I knew that soon enough I would be able to walk up a flight of stairs like a normal person, without a second thought. The threat of disability lifted and flittered away. I was taking my life back.

Chapter Twelve

Fail!

My body was on the fast track to healing. I felt better and better every single day. I was even able to start exercising again right away.

I kept it light at first. The stationary bikes at the gym were my friends. I rode for up to a half hour at a time before I worked my way into to ten or fifteen minutes on the elliptical machines. My toes were still going numb so I couldn't use those pretend skiing machines for too long before the tingling in my feet started to get to me. I followed the advice I had read online for people with auto-immune disorders who are trying to add exercise back into their lifestyles; I went slow and I didn't overdo it. Until I did. Three weeks into the diet, I went for a five-mile hike with some friends at Silver Falls State Park.

It wasn't smart, but I felt so much better that I was sure I could do it. It was, after all, just a long walk in the forest. I walked all day long at work. How much harder could it be? Besides, before my body gave out on me, I used to hike there all the time. I forgot about the inclines and declines, the uneven trail from one waterfall to the next; all the things that would fatigue my recovering muscles and wrench my still healing back. And I forgot how hungry it made me.

I ate breakfast but it was not enough. I took food with me but it wasn't either. Strawberries, jicama soaked in lemon juice, green plantain "fries"—it was a great snack—but I was famished before the hike was over.

To make matters worse, the skies let loose on the last couple of miles. It didn't just rain, it poured. Even with the tree cover, we were drenched. The cold water soaked through my clothes and hair. It didn't take long for the trail to fill with puddles and mud so my shoes soaked through too. By the last mile I was miserable: cold, sopping wet, and starving. My body started to hurt. I felt sick.

And I was tired. Bone tired.

That hike was the most exercise I had done in months. My body ached by the time I got home, paying me back for what I had put it through. At that point I couldn't imagine cutting up sweet potatoes or roasting broccoli. I had yet to figure out what I could eat in a hurry or when I was too drained to cook. I wasn't up for any kind of meal prep. And I was so hungry, so unbelievably hungry. I needed to eat right away.

So, I cheated.

I went to Jack in the Box and ordered an Ultimate Cheeseburger. Looking back over a year later and I haven't had anything like that since, it sounds absolutely disgusting. But I was so hungry that it tasted divine. So salty and gooey. I ordered it without ketchup and mustard, extra mayo. Lots and lots of mayo. I love mayo. I gobbled it down and took a nap on the couch.

Processed cheese. A wheat bun. Seasonings made of who knows what on the meat. Mayo-onion sauce (eggs and processed gunk). One or more of these things brought the ulcers raging back. The next morning, I woke up with holes in my mouth.

Chapter Thirteen

Misdiagnosed, Again

With my work schedule, I couldn't fit in a visit to the clinic until a couple of days later, when the sores were already considerably smaller than when they showed up the day after I ate that fateful cheeseburger. They still hurt and they still looked gross and I knew that it was something in that fast food sandwich that had caused them so I went in anyway, determined to get answers.

I was the last patient of the day; the last patient of the day on a Friday. I don't know why I even bothered. My assigned provider talked about herself and her workload for most of the appointment, then she took one quick look at the sores in my mouth and made her misdiagnosis. Want to guess what she said?

Herpes.

I don't know how I stayed calm. I told her to look at my chart, my tests had always been negative. She looked back only as far as the one that had been cancelled when I saw her colleague about a month prior. She re-ordered it.

She told me it wasn't the bad kind, it was the kind "you get when your mother kisses you on the lips as a baby. It's just type A, one in four adults . . ." *blah blah blah*.

If I've had it since I was a baby why has it never been a problem before?
I bet nobody can guess what she said! It's going to blow your mind!
Stress. Motherfucking stress.

She seriously sat there in her white doctor's coat on her little swivel chair that creaked beneath her and told me that I had holes all over my mouth because stress triggered an immune response by the herpes virus that she claimed had been hiding in my system, undetected by previous blood tests, since I was a baby.

Never mind that, aside from my waning health, that period of my life was one of the least stressful times in my adult life.

I told her about my diet and my slip up, she didn't think it was relevant.

I told her about my joint pain, about how my elbows burned and woke me up at night. I told her about my stiff hands and knuckles, how I constantly dropped my keys and other small objects. She told me it was arthritis.

At 35? At 35 she would have me believe that I was experiencing the symptoms of gerontology? That I had arthritis so bad that I was losing my ability to function? And there was nothing wrong with that? That my rapidly declining health and fitness shouldn't be a reason for concern, why?

I described how I had been crawling out of bed before I went on the diet, how I still woke up stiff and in pain. I explained that my mom had been diagnosed with R.A.

She got mad. Her bitch switch flipped. Where she had been perfectly happy talking about herself for ten of the fifteen-minute appointment, she was not about to listen to my symptoms. I had a whole list of them and she didn't want to hear any. She basically told me I had had a good run, being as healthy as I had up until that point, and that I should just accept my symptoms as inevitable. It was just a part of getting older.

At thirty fucking five?!

I insisted something was wrong.

"Fine," she huffed, "I'll order you an ANA panel, but it's just arthritis."

Nope sorry doc, debilitating arthritis is not something that just happens in the mid-thirties!

The one thing that she was concerned about at that visit was my blood pressure. It was ridiculous, the top number was near 160. My pulse was over 140. But that wasn't why I was there and I wasn't about to walk out of her office with a prescription for blood pressure pills when I knew that my overarching problem was auto-immune.

By the time I got out of the appointment, the lab was closed, so I couldn't go in for bloodwork until Monday. I spent the weekend searching for answers on the internet. I knew it had to be one of the ingredients in the Ultimate Cheeseburger that triggered the flare up in my mouth.

Dairy was the obvious first suspect. For most of my life I would get nauseous and my belly would swell instantly after having milk or soft cheeses, so I naturally thought I might be lactose intolerant. Could the fake, processed cheese in the burger been enough dairy to trigger a reaction?

I didn't find anything online that linked lactose intolerance to the kind of sores I had in my mouth, or the bulk of other symptoms I was experiencing. But there was one ingredient in that cheeseburger that was a much more likely offender.

The bun.

And there was one autoimmune disease that could account for all my symptoms, where others could only be responsible for a few. There was one disease that could explain why my mouth began to clear up within days of going on the Paleo AIP diet, and why the rest of my body's recovery, though slower, was close behind.

Celiac.

Celiac? But that's just a stomach thing, right?

Wrong. So very, very wrong.

It was something I had heard of before, I was aware that it existed, but I had no idea the extent of the damage it could do to a person's body. Celiac is a full-fledged autoimmune disorder that affects the entire body. Its symptoms cover a range that damages just about every system in the body, not just the digestive and intestinal tract.

I had a lot of symptoms spread out among a lot of different autoimmune disorders, but no one disorder accounted for all my symptoms.

Except celiac.

Everything that was wrong with me was listed as a possible symptom of celiac, among hundreds of others. Even things I didn't realize were a part of the disease process, turned out to be symptoms of celiac disease. The erosion of enamel at my gum line was one of them. Where I blamed myself for that, thinking that maybe all the soda I drank had finally caught up with me, it turned out it was all part of the autoimmune mystery.

I called my medical provider back on Monday and asked for a celiac panel to be added to my orders. I didn't really expect it to get included, but it was. I went into the lab and said goodbye to three vials of blood.

.

Chapter Fourteen

Results

My medical provider didn't like the results of my bloodwork. They didn't back her up and she didn't bother calling me to discuss my test results even though there was clearly mild inflammation on my ANA panel and my herpes screen was . . . dun dun dun . . . 100% negative!

I was right, she was wrong, and she did everything she could to stall me out of asking her for answers. She mailed me my results, with a note at the bottom that I should call if I had questions. _IF_ I had questions? Of course, I had questions! How could I not have questions? What would have been the point of having the bloodwork done if I wasn't going to get any answers out of it?

I called, left a message with reception. Her nurse called back, requesting that I call back again. This went back and forth a couple of times until the nurse finally called while I was off from work and able to answer. Just to tell me that if I wanted to discuss my test results I would need to make an appointment and come in to the clinic. So why didn't my provider write that in her note to begin with? Why did she leave instructions for me to call her instead of writing that I should make an appointment in the first place? This phone tag game was a ploy to make me give up and stop bothering her, that much was obvious.

It worked. I rolled my eyes and hung up. Why waste another two hours of my life for a fifteen-minute appointment so she could talk more about herself and her workload?

As far as I was concerned, she didn't know what was wrong with me and she didn't want to do the work to figure it out. She didn't want to play doctor. In other words, she didn't want to do her job. Maybe I was mistaken, but my experiences with her up to that point hardly make me think she was going to sit down and listen to my symptoms and then put any effort into figuring out the cause.

She didn't like me, that much was obvious the two times that I had seen her. First for my back when she assumed I was drug seeking, then when I refused to accept her herpes and arthritis misdiagnosis. She clearly wanted me to leave her alone. I was one of those pesky patients that would force her do something other than get out her prescription pad.

But she was useless, just like the previous providers I had seen. All any of them ever wanted to do was treat the symptoms, whether it was to throw pills at them or tell me to "try and be less stressed out". They never wanted to dig for the root cause that would have made me better years, no decades, ago.

Screw it, I thought. My friend, the physical therapist, had already done way more to help me than any MD or NP I had ever gone to see. Not only had she determined that my symptoms were clearly autoimmune, but she went on to staff my mysterious symptoms with her colleagues. She took my list of symptoms to a naturopath, two nurse practitioners, two surgeons, a neurologist, a PHD physiologist, a PhD neuroscientist, and a registered nurse. While obviously, none of them could diagnose me based on my narrative of symptoms (malpractice anyone?) they were extremely helpful in their responses. The majority agreed that I had something autoimmune going on. Bechet's, R.A., and celiac were mentioned, among others. Most of them also agreed that I should continue with the elimination diet.

My friend also offered to help interpret my bloodwork. I didn't have herpes. Woohoo! While that part of the test results was easy enough to read, stamped with three big NEGATIVEs, it was nice to have a medical professional reiterate that.

My celiac panel was negative, but she explained that could be because, except for the slip up with the Ultimate Cheeseburger, I had been on a gluten free diet for three weeks prior to taking the test. Come to find out, the blood panel is only helpful if the patient is on a gluten containing diet, and even the panel wasn't very accurate. I could retake the test after eating a bunch of gluten based foods, though it still wasn't guaranteed to be accurate.

Mmmm burritos, pizza, beer, cake! Why not?

After how I felt following just one cheeseburger, and how much better I continued to feel the longer I was on the ridiculously strict diet, I chose to continue with the Autoimmune Protocol that was in the process of giving my life back to me instead.

My ANA panel was a little more mysterious than the other two tests. I didn't have the markers for R.A., but I clearly had some mild inflammation. And it could be caused by celiac as my friend explained. She hoped for my sake that it wasn't. Celiac is awful, after all. Awful!

Still, I wasn't discouraged. I would rather have a disease I can control by not eating things than one that I would have to rely on medication to keep at bay. The last thing I wanted was a life full of anti-inflammatories, pain pills, and appointments with more doctors.

Chapter Fifteen

Time for a Challenge

Fast forward a couple of months. I reached my goal—60 days on the elimination diet were up. It was time to start challenging foods to see what I could put back on my plate. I was so excited. There were so many things I missed. Where would I even begin?

With failure, that's where! I failed big time, I did it all wrong.

I didn't mean to. I mean, I knew how I was supposed to do it. Eat a small bite of whatever food I chose to challenge, wait fifteen minutes or so and watch for the return or worsening of autoimmune symptoms, such as: digestive reactions (heartburn, cramps, gas, bloating, vomiting, or diarrhea), mental reactions (such as brain fog, mood swings, anxiety, depression, suddenly feeling overwhelmed by life), symptoms of seasonal allergies (coughing, sneezing, itchy eyes, itchy throat), headaches, arthritis/joint pain, aches and pains in muscles, ligaments, or tendons, and ulcers in the mouth or nose. If symptoms developed, the challenge would be over and the food in question would remain eliminated. If no symptoms developed, I was supposed to eat another small bite and wait fifteen more minutes. Again, if any symptoms reared their ugly heads, the challenge was over and the food in question would stay in the no-no column. If none showed I could eat a still bigger bite, then wait two to three hours and watch for symptoms again. If none developed, I was supposed to eat a full serving of the food in question. Then, because symptoms can delay for a few days, I wasn't supposed to eat any more of the challenged food or challenge any new foods for five to seven days while monitoring for symptoms. If none developed during that time then I could reintroduce the food into my diet and challenge a new food. (https://www.thepaleomom.com/start-here/the-autoimmune-protocol/)

So, while I knew what to do in theory, when I went to put it into practice I went straight off the deep end and attempted my first challenge at a restaurant. See, eating out is something I really, really enjoy. Cooking is tons of fun and all, I really do love it most of the time. And I prefer to feed my family home cooked food. But sometimes food just tastes better when I don't have to make it myself. There's no dicing or slicing or sautéing or pureeing. There's no running to the store for missing ingredients. There's no fielding complaints from kids who wanted ribs or tacos instead. Instead of serving everyone else, someone serves me? Yes, please! And best of all, there's no clean up afterwards.

I hadn't been to a restaurant for the entire 60 days since starting the diet. And as much as I do love to cook, I didn't want to do it three times a day. I couldn't just have cereal for breakfast, remember? I WAS SO SICK OF COOKING ALL THE TIME.

Somehow, I got the idea that I could challenge tomatoes at a restaurant. They only use a small amount in a salad, why not? I would simply order the rest of my food according to the Paleo AIP diet. Before I even left the house, I told myself I was going to be careful and order no this and no that, but by the time I got there I forgot all about how careful I needed to be. I forgot that salads come with cheese and I should have had that 86'd in addition to the croutons. I may have also forgotten to order the oil and vinegar for myself when I ordered ranch for my daughter. And I mean if it's already at the table I might as well use it. I WAS SO SICK OF OIL AND VINEGAR! And oil & lemon . . . and . . . and . . .

We had crab legs too and they would have been fine with the diet except I went all out on the butter. Again, it was already at the table, so I used it. *More butter please!* (I love butter. I love butter and chocolate milk and mayo and I am not ashamed to admit it! Not together, silly.)

There went dairy and eggs.

The one thing I did succeed at ordering correctly? Oyster shooters. *Just lemons.*

This is not how you're supposed to do it. I did it all wrong.

If I had reacted to either the tomatoes (a nightshade), the dairy in the cheese, butter, and ranch, or the eggs (mayo) or potential thickeners in the ranch, I would have no way of knowing which one it was. Nor would I have any way of knowing whether there was more than one culprit. Any symptoms and I would have had no way of knowing which ingredient brought them on. I would have had to hit the reset button on the diet and the food challenges.

The result? I was lucky. Nothing happened. I didn't wake up the next morning with sores in my mouth nor did any develop over the next week. My back didn't seize up and my joints did not feel as though they had caught fire. I continued to heal and feel a little stronger and a little less foggy every day.

Chapter Sixteen

Relief

There should be a word for what I felt when I realized that I would never have many of the world's best foods or most of my own favorites ever again. There probably is and it's probably in German or something.

I wish I had that word, whatever language it is in.

Then another for when I was just grateful that I was not going to end up in a wheelchair with ulcers on my coochie and the kind of eyes people only look into because their parental figures never taught them that it isn't polite to stare.

After passing the oral challenge, in spite of my failed methods, it was obvious what the problem was. I rejoiced, secure in the fact that I didn't have Bechet's or R.A. or Lupus or any of those. Still, I was already mourning doughnuts and beer and pizza and flour tortillas.

Chapter Seventeen

Gluten's Day in Court

It was time to challenge gluten and I was going to challenge the shit out of it. Screw the guidelines. If this was going to be my last time with suave grains that make baked goods so fluffy, I was going to eat as much of it as I could in one sitting.

I went all out. I drove up to Claim Jumpers and ordered a Margherita pizza for dinner and the chocolate chip calzone for desert.

What I really mean is the pizza was just the appetizer to what I was really there for. All that soft baked pizza dough wrapped around gooey chocolate filling with just enough but never too much marshmallow on the inside. All that vanilla ice cream, whip cream, regular and white chocolate chips, chocolate sauce, and fresh mint on the outside.

None of this was wise. Definitely don't do it this way.

I say that but I am a complete hypocrite. I am glad I did it that way, regardless of the consequences. It was my last meal so to speak. And it was amazing!

The cheese on the pizza was melted just right. The crust was perfectly crusty. The tomatoes were perfectly spaced, not too many, not too few. The basil was fresh. I savored it like it was the last pizza I would ever eat.

Fifteen minutes after I ordered it, the chocolate chip calzone appeared. It really did take that long, it said it would on the menu, and the server made sure to point it out as well. It may have taken 'forever' in dining time, but it was well worth the wait.

The dessert was heaven on a plate. The marshmallow was melted with precision. There was a perfect balance of regular chocolate chips and sweeter white chocolate chips. The temperature contrast between the calzone with its gooey melted center and the vanilla ice cream made for a party in my mouth.

The last party a la chocolate chip calzone as it turns out—that much was clear by the time I hit the freeway home. Heartburn raged; my esophagus was on fire; acid lapped at my throat. By the time I pulled into my parking space, I wanted to throw up.

I went straight to bed. Not that I could sleep, I felt way too crappy for that. I just laid there in the fetal position and felt sorry for myself.

And yet I stand by my earlier statement. It was worth it.

The first few times I heard of the chocolate chip calzone, all I could think was, *that sounds disgusting.* A dessert wrapped in pizza dough? No thank you! I was forced to try it. Not kidding. It was ordered by a friend and put in front of me and it smelled like heaven. I had to try a piece.

It was scrumptious! It was chewy and gooey and chocolatey and . . . and . . . I would probably commit human sacrifice if it meant I could eat a chocolate chip calzone without consequence. Or real flour tortillas. Or a glazed donut. Or drink a pint of stout.

Just kidding . . . maybe. I mean, there's got to be some kind of voodoo that would work, right?

When I woke up the next morning my body ached. It was like I had hit rewind on all the healing I had experienced the previous two months. My back was stiff. My elbows burned. My knees hurt. And my stomach? Let's just say I kind of wanted to die. My brother came over for something and asked me why I was walking hunched over. I didn't even realize I was, I just knew that my back hurt as bad as it did before I went on the diet. It took a little longer for the ulcers in my mouth to come back this time, but they did. With a vengeance!

There was no arguing with the oral challenge. It confirmed the obvious. I was both disappointed and grateful. Gluten makes food taste amazing. I love gluten. Why me? But at least I wouldn't have to take Humira for the rest of my life. Or painkillers. I wouldn't end up in a wheelchair or in an assisted living facility. I rejoiced in those facts. Had I been given a choice in the matter I would still choose celiac over any of the other autoimmune diseases that had loomed as possibilities. The great thing about celiac vs. Bechet's, R.A., Crohn's, Sjogren's, Lupus, Psoriasis, etc., is that it is completely controllable. So long as I stay far, far away from gluten, I am fine!

Chapter Eighteen

The Calm and Then the Storm

All I had to do to feel better was stop ingesting gluten, but my medical provider prescribed me muscle relaxers and anti-inflammatories and she sent me to a pain clinic to learn how to live with the pain for the rest of my life instead.

I paid out of pocket for massages and chiropractic adjustments when all I needed to do was cut certain food and drinks from my diet. I spent hundreds if not thousands of dollars trying to alleviate my pain enough to keep working. The chiropractor didn't understand why my back kept getting worse either.

I stretched and I tried to exercise, ignoring the pain as much as I could. I stretched a lot: before I crawled out of bed, after I got out of bed, before I went to work. At work, I would sneak into the office or the walk-in cooler and touch my toes and try to stretch my back out enough to keep going. I stretched my thighs and calves and popped my hips. Every once in a while, someone would walk in on me and their face would say *What the fuck are you doing?* while their lips said, "Oh, sorry."

And because I was willing to try anything to feel better, I went to those classes at the pain clinic, the first half of which were helpful. Yoga and relaxation. It was a little rudimentary but I picked up some helpful poses that helped me pop my back and stretch my spine. But after yoga we were directed to a classroom. I could have done without the class time, since I mostly just sat there wondering, what am I doing here?

I looked around the room. I had nothing in common with anyone. Even then, over a year before I knew celiac was the problem, I knew I was going to get better. I was determined. Long before my friend would bless me with her open ears and open heart and set me on the path to the miracle of healing, I knew I would get better.

When I looked around at my fellow classmates what I saw were a lot of people who owned their pain. It was part of their identity. I would not allow pain to become my identity! I fought it every step of the way.

Every class I listened to the others complain about their bodies. "My pain was so bad last night I didn't sleep a wink. . ." "My pain won't let me do anything anymore . . ." It was a part of them. They complained that their doctors didn't understand. They NEEDED the Vicodin and Percocet. They NEEDED it!

And while I am sure many of them had real diseases and nerve damage that caused very real pain, I was not going to be anything like them. I told myself that was not my future. I would not be like them. Instead of focusing on the pain that racked my body, the muscle spasms that attacked my back, the throbbing in my leg, the aching and burning in my joints, I focused on how much further I could ride my bike, or how kicking a soccer ball against a wall at the park with my daughter had helped stretch and strengthen the muscle in my back that caused me the most grief.

I don't know where it came from, but for once in my life I chose to be positive. And it helped. Maybe it didn't bring me the miracle of healing that I needed, but it brought me a little relief and let me return to some of my previous activities for a few months.

I tried to make the most out of the classes, though most everything was just a refresher of what I already knew. We learned about belly breathing, which I was already doing naturally. We drew pictures of what we would do if we were free of pain. Yup, we got to color in class as if we were kindergartners! We learned about opioid dependence and overdose. That was the one thing that was new to me, but it was useless information. I wasn't there because I had solicited my doctors for pain medication one too many times.

I went until they kicked me out for missing a class (I was stuck on the toilet, thank you celiac) and an appointment with their nurse (thank you, celiac brain fog). The instructor claimed that I had missed two classes, which I hadn't, but my brain was in such a haze that I couldn't recall the last class I had been to so there was no arguing with her. When I got home and went through my notebook I saw the coloring sheet I had done from that second class that I had not actually missed, so I knew I was right. By then it was too late of course.

The instructor said I could enroll in the next set of classes but I didn't see the point. Thus far the workshop felt like a giant waste of gas and time so that I could do a little yoga but mostly listen to people bitch and moan. I decided to move along and focus on exercise, stretching, and meditation on my own. What did I need with a pain clinic meant for people who were flirting with opioid addiction anyway?

Time went on and I thought I was getting some relief from these methods. I thought all the stretching I was doing was working. Never mind that I had to stretch quite a bit before I could even get out of bed, then again once I was out of bed, for a total of a good half hour every morning. Then again throughout my day. Or that I had to exercise for two hours a day and visit a chiropractor and a masseuse bi-weekly for minor results. Every step I took still hurt, just not as much. I felt marginally better.

For once, I was grateful. I was getting my life back. Little by little the pain lessened. I could do more for longer. I could ride my bike. I could play tennis with my daughter and chase her around the jungle gym in short bursts. I was never not in some sort of pain, but it was a lot more manageable for a while.

Of course, there is more, another piece to the puzzle. A piece I didn't even realize at the time. A piece I didn't recognize until a year later when I challenged gluten. The real reason I was feeling better wasn't just the stretching or exercise or all the money I was spending on adjustments and massages. It was a change I had made to my diet.

You see, I had noticed what looked like cavities on a couple of my teeth. The enamel was gone at the gum line. In hindsight, I should have seen a dentist. Maybe they would have diagnosed me correctly. As I found out later, dentists are often the ones who recognize celiac where doctors have failed, and it is because of this type of erosion.

But after that one experience with a dentist who wanted to drill unnecessary holes in my mouth so he could bill my insurance, the last thing I was going to do was see a dentist and get a mouth full of fillings. I turned to the internet instead. I learned all about remineralization diets. Carbs were now my enemy and I cut back on anything high in phytic acid: nuts, seeds, beans, rice, and especially grains.
(https://wellnessmama.com/3650/remineralize-teeth/)

I started to feel better. But I thought it was just because the insane amount of exercise and stretching I was doing was paying off.

Another clue I missed? Just prior to going on the reminiralization diet is when I first started to get patches of canker sores in my mouth. They weren't that bad at first. They certainly weren't anything like the giant holes I would get later that year. I didn't think much of them other than noticing that they were listed as a possible side effect of the anti-inflammatories my medical provider had prescribed for my back, which I immediately stopped taking.

The sores went away. At the time it seemed obvious why, but it was just a coincidence that they healed when I stopped taking the medicine. I didn't have any idea that the sores were actually caused by an autoimmune reaction to gluten and I didn't realize that in drastically cutting out the number of carbs I was taking in, I had inadvertently cut the amount of gluten I was consuming way down.

I thought my mouth was better because I stopped taking the pills that didn't seem to be helping anyway. And my body was hurting less because of all the exercise and stretching, right? It made sense, but it wasn't the case.

In the fall, I gave up the remineralization diet and the exercise. I was working three jobs (long story) and I still had the internship at the brewery. With no time to cook, let alone energy, this was when I became dependent on fast food. And when my health started to go downhill faster than ever.

By late winter 2015 my back was seizing up worse than it ever had before. My toes were going numb. So were my hands and parts of my face. It felt like a nerve was being pinched somewhere in my spine.

Work was torture. I hated everyone. The drive home was pure agony. After eight to ten hours on my feet my right leg would cramp and spasm the entire drive. Every time I had to use the brake an extra surge of pain shot up through my back.

My elbows burned. My hands were stiff and I dropped things constantly. I dropped my keys at least once every time I went to unlock my own front door. There were scabs all over my scalp. I was anxious and angry and couldn't think straight. My brain felt like it was tucked into a thick gray fog.

The sores in my mouth were back with a vengeance. It wasn't just patches of white spots that looked like canker sores anymore either. Some of the ulcers got to be almost as big as a dime. Had I noticed the correlation between returning to a carb laden diet (and therefore gluten) and the resurgence of the ulcers back then, I could have saved myself over half a year of needless suffering.

Chapter Nineteen

Easier Said Than Done

Once I knew what was wrong with me I was happy to give up the limitations of the Auto Immune Protocol for the relative freedom of the celiac diet. I was relieved to know I could have dairy, nightshades, beans, nuts, and everything else I cut out—all of it— except gluten.

Easier said than done.

And by that I do not mean willpower. That part is easy enough. I know what will happen if I put a piece of bread in my mouth or try to nibble on a donut or make a quesadilla with a flour tortilla instead of a corn one. I know what will happen if I drink a beer. I know what will happen if I eat a dish made with soy sauce or a rue. So I don't. I dream about it on occasion. Mid-bite I realize what I have done and I am filled with dread. Then I wake up. This last time I was eating coconut shrimp in my dream. I don't even like coconut shrimp.

When the body reacts violently to a food it is easy enough to purposefully not eat it. The problem is what I might ingest on accident and without knowing.

Many people are under the mistaken impression that the surge in gluten free menus makes it easier for people with celiac to eat out. If anything, the opposite is true. The vast majority of restaurants prepare their gluten free menus on the same equipment as their regular ones. And with so many people on fad diets, restaurants are remiss to take any precautions. Over and over I've been told, *yes, we have a gluten free menu, no we don't do anything to protect people with food allergies, we're not equipped for that.* Then what is the point to the gluten free menu? How is it supposed to work for people who can't have gluten when it only takes an 1/8 of a teaspoon of flour to cause malabsorption in most of us?

Sometimes there is a warning right on the menu. Sometimes there isn't. Sometimes the menus are 100% gluten free. Sometimes they have ingredients that whoever developed the menu assumed were gluten free, but they are not. I learned that one the hard way and make my own cocktail sauce at the table in most restaurants.

Oregon was recently rated the number one state to be gluten free in. I laughed out loud when I heard that. In the city where I lived I can count the number of restaurants that will take special precautions on one hand. Surely, this designation was for people who are gluten free by choice, not necessity. That or it must impossible to eat out in the other 49 states. I guess I better be grateful!

Menus aren't the only place gluten is hiding. It is everywhere. And it's not just the obvious wheat, rye, and barley either. Durum, emmer, semolina, farina, spelt, farro, and graham are all off limits too, as they come from wheat. As do most grains with wheat as part of the name (wheatberries, Khorasan wheat, einkorn wheat, but not buckwheat which is a totally different grain). Wheat starch (unless processed in a way to remove gluten). Triticale. Brewer's Yeast. Malt. Yes, that's right, malted milk shakes and malt vinegar are chock full of gluten! Even flours that are naturally gluten free, such as corn flour, can be contaminated in the field or factory.

It should be obvious that any foods made from gluten containing grains have gluten in them. It should be, but most people aren't used to thinking of their food that way. I don't even know how many times I've been flabbergasted as I explained to someone that just because they didn't put flour in a pasta dish, that doesn't make it gluten free.

"It's not wheat, it's spaghetti."

Shaking my head.

Pastas, noodles, breads, pastries, and baked goods, as a rule, are also full of gluten. Gnocci may be made from potato flour, but some wheat flour is still used. The same is true of egg noodles. Rice and mung bean noodles, on the other hand, are naturally gluten free (assuming they are not contaminated in the factory or cooking process). Cornbread almost always includes wheat flour. Falafel may be primarily chickpeas, but there is often still a tiny bit of white flour used in most recipes. I found that out the hard way in Nicaragua. Yes, falafel in Nicaragua—this is a beautiful diverse world we live in. Crackers, cereal, and granola, unless gluten free, are not safe either. Plenty of cereals made from rice and corn contain malt syrup, for example.

More examples of foods that should be obvious: breakfast foods like pancakes, waffles, and crepes, breaded foods such as fried chicken and tempura. Flour tortillas are also a given, but corn tortillas can contain trace amounts of gluten from field and factory contamination, or from being cooked or heated on the same surface as flour ones. Soups, sauces, and gravies often contain gluten because flour is used as a thickener. Salad dressings aren't safe either due to additives. Soy sauce may sound fine for those without a soy allergy, but wheat is actually a major ingredient (tamari is wheat free soy sauce). The original British recipe for Worcestershire is made with soy sauce and malted vinegar, as are many generic versions of the sauce.

Fermented and malted adult beverages are unsafe unless certified gluten free. Liquor, on the other hand, is okay unless some sort of gluten containing flavoring is added after the distillation process. Celiacs rejoice and feel free to drink all the sweet rye vodka you want! (I mean, drink responsibly . . .)

When it comes to pre-packaged and prepared foods, gluten can be in almost anything. Chicken, for example, is naturally gluten free. But if it comes with a spice rub or any type of flavoring added, the potential for gluten is there. Soups may or may not be made with a roux which is made from wheat flour. French fries are often coated in flour. Even when they're not, if they are cooked in a fryer that is used for any breaded or gluten containing items, they are not celiac safe.

Candy, granola, and chips can all contain gluten in the form of flour or malt flavoring. Even ice cream can have it, either because of the flavor, such as cookies'n'cream, or because of contamination from being processed on the same equipment. Processed meats often contain wheat and other grain products as fillers. If there is an ingredient list, I have to read it. Just looking for the Contains Wheat warning isn't enough either. Remember, rye, barley, and wheat derivatives are just as problematic.

The one time I tried to play loose by the rules, I got burned. I ate a lot of stewed chicken in Belize only to feel like absolute shit by the time I got to Guatemala. The dish looked safe enough. The sauce was too thin to have any flour in it and, I thought, too red to have any of the liquid offenders like soy sauce. Turns out it's made with both soy sauce and Worcestershire. Or Salsa Inglesa as it says on labels south of the Mexican-American border. And it has a clear warning: contains wheat. It may not have been a ton of gluten relative to something like a piece of cake, but it was enough to bring on a wave of anxiety and sadness, make my back, hips, and elbows ache, and turn the chilly mountain air bone cold in Antigua. Until that incident I didn't realize what an intense effect a little bit of gluten had on my ability to tolerate the cold.

It's not just foods either. Gluten is used in all sorts of products that can be accidently ingested. Or on purpose, if you've got a kid who puts on flavored lip gloss just so they can lick it off. Or one that eats play-dough. See celiac.org for a more comprehensive list of food and non-food items that may contain gluten. No list is exhaustive however. When you have celiac, you have to verify that every product is gluten free before putting it in or near your mouth.

Chapter Twenty

Reactions

"So how much gluten can you have exactly?" Yup, that's a serious question people ask. It's completely innocent but it makes me laugh every time as I want to reply, 'I don't know, how many peanuts can someone with a peanut allergy eat?'

None. The blatantly obvious answer is none.

A dear friend and regular at the bar I tended told me I could probably eat gluten just fine in less developed countries. He was serious. He thought I would be able to avoid an autoimmune reaction if I ate wheat outside of the United States. My laughter was not appreciated, but I couldn't help it, it was a hilarious statement. The fact that he was so serious made it even funnier.

It has been a learning process, finding humor in people's reactions. Sometimes, I make the mistake of letting it annoy me, especially when someone who doesn't have a clue what they are talking about tries to commiserate.

The following section is something I wrote before I realized how ungrateful I was being for my healing. I had taken on an attitude of victimhood. I was tired of having to ask so many questions at restaurants. I was tired of gluten free menus aimed at fad dieters instead of those of us with an actual disease. I was tired of not being able to just go out and eat like a normal person.

I forgot to be thankful for my own good fortune My body wouldn't destroy itself so long as I was careful about what I put in it. I wouldn't end up in a wheelchair or dependent on others to care for me. Disability was no longer in my future. But at the time, I was taking it all for granted. Hence, the tone of the following section on commiseration. I decided to include it because other people with celiac can relate. If you find, whether from an elimination diet or a biopsy of your intestines, that you are banned from gluten for life, this is the sort of stuff that is out there. These are the sort of things people say even with the best intentions.

"Oh my god, I know exactly what you mean!"

No. No you don't hipster girl . . . I stopped myself, I was being judge-y. She continued. "I'm gluten free too! It's gotten sooooo bad that I can't even drink whisky anymore because of the breakouts. They're awful!"

No. No. No. And, no! There is nothing worse at a restaurant (well besides being glutened) than a "gluten intolerant" server who tries to commiserate!

I smiled and bit my tongue. One—the gluten peptide is too big to make it through the distillation process. Sorry, but unless you're soaking a piece of bread in your whisky it is naturally gluten free. Two—she breaks out? Was she kidding me?! Was she seriously comparing a few pimples to an autoimmune disease that puts me in the fetal position with nausea, sends my blood pressure through the roof, makes the world feel like it is falling down around me, destroys my muscles and joints, and was well on its way to taking my teeth?!

It is human I guess, to try and relate to another's pain. But it's also rude and insulting when someone doesn't know what they are talking about, when they try to relate to something they only pretend to understand.

It's even worse when friends do it. Especially the ones who have made lifestyle choices that have caused their own supposed misery. And of course, Facebook can be the worst. I made the mistake of posting a bitch and moan session about gluten free menus and cross contamination. A "vegetarian" friend commented in agreement: "OMG I totally know what you mean. It makes me so sick when they cook my veggie burger on the same grill as hamburger."

No! Sorry my friend, but you don't know.

I tried to call her out as politely as possible: "Being grossed out by something is hardly the same thing as an autoimmune reaction."

She commented back, insisting that it made her physically ill.

I'm sorry, but bullshit.

Another friend jumped in to defend her. Not a mutual friend either, but maybe she is a vegetarian too so I can only guess that was her motivation. She pointed out that long term vegetarians often do get sick if they eat meat.

Okay I will concede that as a possibility. If they are a real vegetarian who takes a bite of actual meat, not just get a little hamburger dust on their veggie patties. Still, I was a real vegetarian for five years but when I went back to eating meat I don't recall any stomach discomfort beyond my normal (of course, with undiagnosed celiac I was in a constant state of intestinal discomfort, but it had nothing to do with meat). There was no substantial worsening of the constant nausea, stomach cramps, constipation, diarrhea, or constipated diarrhea that I was already experiencing. And I went full out, chowing down on seafood, chicken, and red meat when I gave up the vegetarian lifestyle. Then again, I was never a full-on vegan. I still got animal proteins from dairy and eggs. But so did this friend with her supposed reaction to hamburger contamination. And her body was already used to processing animal proteins from chicken too. See where I am going with this?

I didn't respond to the second friend. I was pissed and there was no way that I could without offending someone and probably burning bridges I didn't want to burn. I could hardly explain to her on a public forum that in this case, the person in question wasn't even a full-on vegetarian. Sorry, not sorry but eliminating red meat alone does not make one a vegetarian.

Whether it is vegetarianism or gluten free as a personal preference, everyone is entitled to their lifestyle choices. BUT it is just straight up rude to try and compare the results of said choices to someone else's food allergy or auto-immune disease.

See what I mean? I was being completely ungracious. Neither of these ladies meant me any harm. And while I thought they were too focused on "me, me, me" to hear what I was saying, I was too focused on me, me, me to be grateful for my health.

It is up to each of us to learn not to react. Situations like these will arise because people sincerely believe that they are suffering from the same issues. They don't mean any harm. They do not intend to be rude. Nothing positive is accomplished by getting angry and annoyed.

How could I have dealt with these situations more positively? First and foremost, by approaching each of these situations with grace. Instead of focusing on how terrible I had it, I could have recognized that we are each fighting our own battles. Instead of seeing their stories as competing with mine, I could have seen each of these ladies as having their own struggles and shown them compassion. After all, what right did I have to expect compassion if I wasn't willing to give it back without judgement?

Ah, judgement! Guilty as charged. Even before I had the slightest clue about what was going on with my body I would get annoyed with people I deemed fakers. Between gigs as a bartender I occasionally took jobs as a server. Why? I have no idea. I can't stand waiting tables. Talk about stress.

Anyway, I worked at a couple of different places with gluten free menus and I would get so annoyed with people who would say they couldn't have gluten but would then proceed to order something that wasn't gluten free and tell me, "It's okay, it doesn't bother me."

Whaaaaat?

The kitchen at one of these restaurants would take extra precautions for a customer who told us they were allergic to gluten. What was the point of those precautions if they were going to order French fries with their gluten free burger?

"Our fryer isn't gluten free," I explained to one customer. The fries were just sliced potatoes, true, but the fryer was used to cook any number of battered items. It was, to put it simply, a celiac nightmare.

"That's okay," she smiled. "I'm fine with that."

She was fine with that? She was willing to pay $2 extra for a gluten free bun, she was willing to make our kitchen take extra precautions with her burger, but then she was "fine" with fries cooked alongside battered onion rings and the like?

I don't think I bothered entering her food as special request. She got her special bun, but I wasn't about to make the kitchen do extra work. And while she didn't need those extra precautions for her "allergy", I was wrong to judge her. I was wrong to get annoyed with her. I was wrong to let myself react instead of being gracious.

When we react, we hurt ourselves. I put that negativity out into the universe, is it any wonder that I have received it back now that I am on the other side of the table so to speak?

Chapter Twenty-One

Glutened, Again

Imagine a "nut-free menu" prepared on the same equipment as nuts. Or with pesto featured prominently among its entrees because whoever designed the menu didn't realize the yummy green sauce contains pine nuts. Ridiculous, right?

I'm being facetious of course. Nut allergies can kill right away, whereas celiac kills over time. Its seriousness is not as immediate. If it were there probably wouldn't be special menus to begin with. There would be allergen warnings posted on menus and at entrances instead. Shafts of wheat would be etched on glass doorways where they would loom over the handles. Airlines would have to restrict their snacks when a celiac passenger is on board. How embarrassing would that be? A bag of flour would send a portion of the population running. Can you imagine? "Wait! No don't open that bag . . ." *croak *lights out *curtains *fin *That's All Folks!

The fact that this is not my reality gives me so many reasons to be grateful. I can sit next to someone while they eat a sandwich without consequence; assuming they don't rub their sandwich all over my food. And if they did? The consequences for me still pale in comparison to what would happen to someone suffering from an extreme nut allergy whose dining companion breathed peanut dust all up in their face. I am not going to die from a little contamination. Yes, it might make me feel like shit, it might put holes in my mouth and make my body ache, but I'm not going to die. No one is going to have to shove an epi-pen into my thigh because the taqueria cooked my corn tortillas on the same flat top as the flour ones. That alone is a reason to rejoice.

Yes, it sucks biting into something and knowing it isn't right, but I'm not going to keel over from it. Even if a piece gets stuck in my teeth and finds its way into my digestive tract after I spit the bulk of the offending food out, I will live.

How would such a thing happen, you might wonder. Why would I think something was safe only to spit it out in the trashcan? Trusting other people to read labels for me that's how!

One night at work one of the cooks had a special kind of Twix Bar, a limited-edition flavor or something. He insisted that it was awesome and I had to try it. He gave me half. I gave him the side eye as I took the candy but he insisted that he had read the label.

Now this is someone who had just gotten out of a long-term relationship with someone afflicted by celiac, so I trusted him. He had prepared her food for years and knew what the no-noes were. He had prepared my food at work as well without issue. I trusted him.

I bit in. I chewed. Nope. No way there wasn't gluten in it. Still he had promised that he read the label so I didn't spit right away. I held it in my mouth, just in case it was safe, (it did taste good after all) while I dug the wrapper out of the trash. Right at the end of the ingredients, in bold letters, it read: Contains Wheat.

I spit the masticated Twix bar in the trash. I spit again. Then again. I rinsed my mouth with water and spit some more. I dug at my teeth with my fingernails, then a toothpick. I showed him the label.

"I thought it was nuts you couldn't have!" All I can say is that boy must have been high. So high! He knew better. He knew he knew better too.

All I could do was laugh. "You tried to kill me!" I exaggerated.

If it had been a nut allergy that plagued me and those were peanut M&Ms, yeah, but I wasn't really going to die. So, I laughed. He laughed. It was a great near miss. I got all of it out of my mouth and luckily I didn't end up getting sick.

The funniest part about all of this was that this same cook had been there to witness an even worse case of label reading failure not long prior. Or rather total lack of label reading. I had mentioned how I wished I had some jerky but then went on to complain that most jerky is made with soy sauce so I couldn't have it. One of my good customers heard the first part but not the second part and rushed out to get me some jerky.

What a sweetheart, right? That's one of the great things about working in the neighborhood dive bar; the customers become not only friends but almost like family. They know we can't leave the bar so many of them will go get us snacks or other goodies. I've even had regulars run to the dispensary for me since it would close long before the end of my shift. *Shhhh don't tell!*

Anyway, I assumed he had heard the second part of the conversation and had checked the label. Don't assume. Assumptions and celiac do not go together, even when people have the best of intentions. I ate a few pieces and shared the bag with the same cook who went on to feed me the gluten-full candy bar a couple of weeks later.

After the customer left I thought, you know, I really should have read that label first. What's that thing they say about good intentions? The road to hell . . . or the toilet, in my case . . .

I flipped over the package. Soy sauce. It wasn't one of the top ingredients, but it was still there. Followed by the allergen warning: Contains Wheat. I showed the cook and he went wide eyed, "Oh shit, how much did you eat?"

Not much, but as we've established, any is too much.

"So how much gluten can you have exactly?"

I don't know, how many peanuts can someone with a peanut allergy eat?

"You should try to throw up," he said. "I'll watch the bar."

And that's how I ended up in the alley behind my job with my finger down my throat.

We both got a good laugh out of it. Yet only a couple weeks later he was trying to feed me more wheat! But what was I going to do, get mad? I could have. We do choose our own reactions after all. Neither one of them meant to poison me. They were just trying to be nice.

Lesson learned, I always read my own labels now.

Laughter really is the best medicine. Especially when it comes to celiac, since there literally is no medicine. The only treatment is: "Don't eat that!"

I am learning that there is no point in getting angry over menus geared towards fad dieters, just as there is no point in getting upset when someone gives me something I can't have by accident or because they forgot. Do I remember everyone's allergies and intolerances? Hell no. I know my best friend can't have some sort of nightshade, but I don't remember whether it is tomatoes, bell peppers, or eggplant. Does that make me a bad person? Of course not! Would she get pissed at me if I offered her something with the offending nightshade? Don't be silly.

Chapter Twenty-Two

Irony Anyone?

There is irony in my disease, and I do not mean because I can no longer enjoy my favorite foods. That whole human sacrifice thing? Yeah, I could really go for some fish tacos right now! I jest, I jest. No, really.

What I mean is that there is irony in how the puzzle of my illness first came together. Over beer. Yummy, delicious beer full of barley and wheat and rye, the three main offenders. My doctor friend and I had met at a tap house just like we had on several occasions. Like most Oregonians, tap houses and breweries were among my favorite places to chill in the Pacific Northwest, second only to the top of a mountain. (Okay, okay, butte, but mountain sounds so much more majestic!)

There were probably thirty beers on tap, something for everyone. I think I was drinking something dark that night. Probably a stout, or a full-bodied porter if there weren't any stouts on draft. Or maybe it was a Hefeweizen. Either way, between sips, or more likely gulps, I complained about the doctor I had just seen and told my friend about my symptoms. The symptoms that it would turn out were caused by the very thing I was enjoying!

It's been over a year and a half since my last beer. I know exactly what it was too. Bridgeport's IPA. I had bought a six pack just before I learned about the Paleo AIP diet. It took me a couple of days to finish it off but when the pack was gone, that was it. I didn't know it at the time but I would never have another real beer again.

Yes, there is gluten free beer, but I am not exactly eager to give it a try. For the most part, gluten free foods pale in comparison to the real deal. Gluten free pizza is not fluffy like regular pizza or even crunchy like 80's style pizza. It's just kind of chewy. Don't get me wrong, I am happy it exists as an option, but I don't eat nearly as much pizza as I used to. Or pasta, or bread. Gluten free bread is pretty freaking awful.

Now I have read that it is possible to breakdown the chain of amino acids that form gluten by fermenting sourdough bread for over 90 days, but that means the actual dough, not just the starter, so I haven't had the chance to test out this theory. Someday I will and if it works, well, I think I might just cry tears of joy all over the hundreds of loaves I will proceed to ferment and bake. Three months may be a long time to wait for bread, but it will so be worth it for a grilled cheese sandwich. I love grilled cheese sandwiches. Love them! They used to be a mainstay in my diet. Sourdough bread, tomatoes, onions marinated in red wine vinegar, a little mayo, and smoked Havarti; my mouth is watering right now! Or fresh mozzarella with tomatoes and basil, a little balsamic reduction on the side to dip it in. It's just not the same on gluten free bread. But I digress . . .

Even more ironic than the puzzle of my illness coming together over the very thing that was making me sick? I was finishing up an internship at a nano brewery in Portland, a city that is world renowned for its breweries, when my health started going downhill fast. Yes, I was training to be a brewer. How is that for irony?

I started out making beer at home, five gallons at a time. I loved experimenting with different types and flavors. My best batch ever was a spicy chocolate stout. It was divine! I never tested the alcohol content in my homebrew, but I am guessing that it came out around ten percent. I was even a little wobbly after just one 22-ounce bottle. The combination of cacao and chilis created a feeling above and beyond your normal alcohol buzz. It imparted the beer with a euphoria that a few people even compared it to snorting a line of cocaine. Had I been able to continue in the brewing industry I don't doubt that that beer would have been my mark on the world of fermentation.

For almost a year, I spent a day or two at the brewery every week, kegging and bottling beer, cleaning out fermenters, and assisting with brewing as I learned more and more about my favorite adult beverage. I applied for entry level positions at breweries around the state. I had a couple of interviews, one at a well-known craft brewery and another at a smaller up-and coming brewery that no one had heard of yet but whose beer the bar I was working at put on draft not six months later.

At the time, I was sorely disappointed when neither brewery offered me employment, and no more brewers called to grant me interviews. Why didn't anyone want to hire me? I had excellent references. My boss at the brewery told me I was the best intern he had ever had.

I was sure it was because I was girl, and a small one at that. There was no way I could dead lift kegs twice my size, but I also felt like the boys didn't want to let me in their club house.

Eventually my body hurt too much and my brain was too foggy to continue looking for work in the industry. I gave up. While at the time I was angry, bitter even, now I know it was for the best. How horrible would it have been if I had taken a job across state only to find out that the product I was creating was destroying me? You can't brew if you can't taste test your own product. Tasting is integral to the process. I am now eternally grateful to every head brewer who tossed my resume aside, regardless of their reason.

And now that I can see the irony in all of it, well the whole ordeal is kind of funny. The career I wanted would have killed me. Thankfully outside forces stepped in and saved me from making a huge mistake.

Chapter Twenty-Three

Gone Baby, Gone

Brewing wasn't the only thing I had to give up. From exercise to friendships, undiagnosed celiac had a profound impact on my life.

I loved to run. My feet hitting the ground in rhythm with my breathing. In, in, out, in, in, out. Right, left, right, left, right left. My face red, dripping with sweat. My muscles striving for just another quarter mile, exploding in an all-out sprint. I don't know how to jog. I mean I get the concept, but I don't like moving that slow unless I'm walking. So, I run until I am out of breath, then I walk huffing and puffing, until I am ready to run again. Other runners probably think I'm weird but I don't care. Pushing my respiratory system to capacity, my muscles to the failing point, especially in that final sprint, it all gives me a sense of euphoria that I can't even pretend to describe.

Unfortunately, running also jarred my lower back and left it stiff and in worse pain than before. I couldn't do it anymore. I didn't have a choice. I had to give it up.

Running was the first thing to go when the effects of celiac started to branch out beyond my stomach, when they started breaking down the rest of my body. From the time I gave it up, it would be almost five years before I would be able to run again.

Next to go was tennis, especially the brand that I enjoyed. I have never played regular tennis, I don't even know how. Instead, what I played with friends was something we liked to call "Get it Bitch tennis". The rules are simple. Or rather, the rule, which is the name of the game. Bitch better hit the ball. No matter what. There was no out of bounds. If it was a double court then the second court was included in that rule. I mean we tried to keep it in one court even if no one was playing on the other one, but if the ball happened to get smacked into the wrong court than we better hustle our butts after it as it was still very much fair game. It was quite the challenge when there were three players and it was two against one, with each of us taking a turn being the one to run back and forth full court after the ball while the other team shared responsibility for their side.

Get it Bitch was a great way to spend time with friends. It was free except for when we hit the balls into oblivion and had to buy new ones. The public courts weren't the greatest, but they weren't the worst. Most of them were surrounded by chain link fence. In our eagerness to hit the ball, everyone probably crashed into the chain link more than once. Most of the courts were blacktop, with cracks filled in by grass and tree roots poking up along the edges. The boundary lines were generally faded away but that didn't matter, we didn't use them anyway. There was a clay court with weathered nets the neighborhood kids liked to climb and swing on. It suffered the same results of age and lack of maintenance as the others. But at least it had a net—there was one court where chain link stood in for the net. Still, even that one was awesome. It was there and it was free and it provided hours of entertainment and exercise.

It was some of the most fun I have had as an adult, but Get it Bitch had to go.

I couldn't run. I couldn't swing the racket. I couldn't do anything. I couldn't even concentrate on the game.

Oregon boasts some pretty fantastic hiking, including some awesome day hikes within an hour's drive of where I lived. There are old growth forests, ghost towns, waterfalls, a "suspension bridge" that isn't at all the cool kind of suspension bridge that I am used to seeing (but at least there is a nice hike that most visitors don't bother with), and it's all nearby. I hiked rain or shine. With a friend, my kids, or by myself. Until I couldn't anymore.

In-line skating—it's not just a 90s trend anymore and, it's tons of fun. Also, great exercise for the butt and legs, so there's that. Until my muscles became too tight and racked with spasms, my back too stiff to skate safely anymore. Then that was gone too.

The bike was the last to go. And it wasn't even because I couldn't ride it. That was the one exercise I could still do with minimal extra pain. It was the bike rack that did me in. There weren't any bike trails near my home and the combination of my less than stellar cycling skills and the scary number of drivers who don't appear to be paying the least bit attention to anything moving except other cars meant that, yes, I needed a bike rack. And, to get my bulky cruiser onto the rack, I had to negotiate it over two bars just right. It had to fit just so and the bike was heavy. It hadn't been a problem when I bought the bike, but it turned into one over time.

It's kind of funny how slow things like that happen; so slow that I did not notice just how bad off I was until one day I woke up and wondered 'when did I get like this?' I couldn't pinpoint any one point in time but I realized that I have been in pain to one degree or another for all my recent memory.

See why I was pissed when my doctor accused me of not exercising enough? And yes, it was an accusation. It was not a question. She never once asked me about my exercise habits nor abilities. She accused me of not exercising as if I had a choice in the matter; as if I hadn't pushed myself to go as hard as I could manage for as long as I could bear; as if simply not exercising could cause the sort of pain that leaves someone crying on the floor while they wait for their Epsom salt bath in hopes of a little relief. I couldn't even walk my dog, I was in tears after walking my daughter to school in the morning, but all I needed was a little exercise, right?

Chapter Twenty-Four

Becoming Who I Don't Want to Be

I was no longer any fun at the park with my daughter either. Where we used to kick a soccer ball or hit tennis balls off the wall in the covered area, play hopscotch, and chase each other on the jungle gym, all I could do at one point was hope there would be other kids there for her to play with while I just sat there and counted the minutes until we could leave. Because even just sitting there hurt. Trips to the park were short and we went less and less often the more my muscles tightened and joints ached.

I felt like a terrible mother and I was. More and more if I wasn't at work I was trying to rest. Being in pain all the time is exhausting. So is insomnia. Which means I wasted a lot of time trying to sleep. Actually falling asleep and staying asleep—well that was a whole different story. When I wasn't trying to sleep, I had no patience and I couldn't remember anything. My temper flared. To this day my son is convinced I don't listen to him because there was about a six-month period there where everything went in one ear and out the other (of course as a teenager he's been guilty of the same for many, many years but I digress). As I mentioned earlier, I turned to fast food and readymade meals more and more. I was feeding my kids junk on top of not having any energy to spend time with them.

I wrote stuff down to remind myself and then proceeded to forget where I had written what. I missed appointments.

I was a hot mess.

I struggled to keep writing despite the fog that had taken over my brain. My output was pitiful, both in quality and quantity. I stared at the screen on my laptop. I couldn't focus. It took me a long time to write a little bit, and even it would need some heavy-duty rewrites.

My social life was affected. Not only was I no longer able to meet friends for a hike or some Get it Bitch tennis, or have any energy to meet for drinks on my day off (if I had one) but my attitude was shit too. I was negative and angry all the time. I was no fun. People didn't want to be around me and I don't blame them. I wouldn't have wanted to be around me either. I lost a couple of long term friends during this time. Burnt those bridges right up. On a positive note, I am better off without those particular individuals in my life. They weren't exactly the healthiest friendships to begin with. Silver lining, eh?

What about dating? Ha-ha, ha-ha, ha-ha. That can't be a serious question. I mean look at my track record so far. I was tired and angry and mean, why would anyone want to date me? And if I couldn't manage exercise because of the pain in my back and joints, how would I manage sex? The idea is laughable.

My life was in the shitter. I took my frustration out on others. Between the pain in my body and the fog in my head, it was impossible to have any sort of social life, and my family life wasn't any better off.

Chapter Twenty-Five

Meal Time

Discovering that gluten was the source of my problems was a miracle. My body healed and I could return to most normal activities. Most.

There is still one aspect of my social life that celiac will always affect: meal time.

Think about it, eating is a very social activity. Families eat together. Friends eat together. When you are dating someone, you eat together. Going out to eat was one of my favorite social activities whether I went with my family or met friends for drinks and appetizers. Barbecues, picnics, potlucks, these are all social activities that are limited by celiac.

When I first went on the elimination diet that returned my quality of life to me I had to turn down every invitation extended to me that involved food. With such a limited diet, I couldn't realistically eat out or go over to someone else's house for a meal. I ate at home or I brought my own food to work to prepare. The bar I was working in at the time provided us with free meals, but I couldn't take full advantage of that benefit since the menu consisted of burgers, sandwiches, and breaded fried foods. I worked with it as best I could. I ate hamburger patties with grilled onions and mushrooms. I made salads with lettuce, cucumber, and onions when I forgot to bring arugula and berries. If I worked the day shift I had to make sure I cooked my food before anything was ordered; before the grill was coated in vegetable shortening and bread crumbs. If I worked the night shift I had to wait until after the grill had been scrubbed clean and then spot clean it when I was done.

Working in a dive bar, it was rare to get an actual meal break. For most of my shift I would be the only one there, which meant if I forgot to bring food I had to make do with what was available. I got sick of hamburger patties and dressed down salads real quick. I stared at the cherry tomatoes and wished I could have just one, but I was committed to the diet and healing my leaky gut, so I resisted.

As a bartender, my food was on display for every customer to comment on and judge. There was no break room, no place where I could eat away from customers. Depending on how busy it was I either took bites behind the bar, between serving customers, or I sat at the bar and ate there. Even if there was a cook on duty to take my place behind the bar, there was nowhere to escape comments and questions about the food I ate.

I did a lot of explaining during those 60 days on the elimination diet. It didn't bother me at the time. I felt a million times better. I felt human again and I was thankful for the diet because it had given me my life back, even if coworkers and customers alike made fun of the plantains I would bring in to sauté. They joked about the *huge banana* and how it was too ripe. "Are you really going to eat that? You should just make banana bread. You can't eat it like that." Or, "What's wrong with your banana? Why is it so big? It looks rotten."

I just shook my head and laughed as I explained that the black on its skin meant it would be sweet instead of starchy. "It's not a banana, it's a plantain," I clarified. "It's supposed to be that size and color."

"What's a plantain?"

I would cook it up and offer it to the curious customer. It felt good to introduce people to healthy foods they wouldn't otherwise encounter and watch the surprise on their face when they bit into it and discovered that, yes, this sautéed fruit like thing really was delicious. Most of them were shocked to watch me cut up and cook what they were convinced was the ugliest banana they had ever seen.

With the oral challenges completed, and all but one of the food groups I had excluded allowed back in my diet, I thought the questions and comments would wane. That was naïve. People continued to look over my shoulder or across the bar at my plate and talk about how I was eating rabbit food. Even if there was a steak on my plate, the load of vegetables overrode the meat and made it rabbit food apparently. I was constantly asked if I was on a low-carb diet. Or told that I shouldn't be on a low-carb diet since I needed some meat on my bones anyway. (Why, oh, why does everyone think they have the right to comment on a woman's weight, whether she is deemed too thick or too thin?)

I let it get to me after a while. I got sick of explaining my health and diet and what celiac is almost every single day and to nearly every single customer who happened to be around when I was trying to eat. I got annoyed with their comments and judgement. I wondered why people felt entitled to share their opinions on my food when I never openly criticized their trans-fat drenched orders or requests for more and more ranch. (I swear people in Oregon use food as spoons for ranch. They would probably order pints of it to drink if it were offered on tap.)

I was not gracious. I reacted and let other people's ignorance, no matter how innocent it was, affect me. I was quick to lose the gratitude I had previously felt for my healing. I began to feel cheated.

Even though a celiac diet is not anywhere near as intense as the Paleo AIP diet, I still must be careful about going to barbecues. Spice mixes and sauces can be riddled with gluten. A lot of people cook their meats with beer and soy sauce, so I worry about contamination with good reason.

Picnics and potlucks aren't any better. The vast majority of foods are unsafe. People will tell me that there isn't any gluten in their dish, but they don't know what gluten is. They don't know that wheat, rye, and barley doesn't mean just bread. They don't know that a little flavoring from malt vinegar or soy sauce or the wrong brand of Worcestershire could do me in. They don't understand that any processed food is suspect. Some people get offended and assume I am just a food snob. Others feel sorry for me and offer me a beer, which of course I can't drink.

Gone are the days of meeting friends for drinks and appetizers. Even ordering a Bloody Mary means I have to bug the bartender with questions about their mix. And those appetizers? Nope, can't have them.

I've already discussed gluten free menus and the few restaurants I trust to control for contamination. Now imagine trying to date someone who doesn't have celiac. It's one thing when you are already with someone who cares about you when you find out you have an autoimmune reaction to a food that is everywhere and in just about everything. It's a whole other thing to try and get to know someone when they can't take you to any old restaurant, let alone their favorite. People bond over food so trying to get to know someone when you have a food allergy can be ridiculous. The last guy who asked me out for lunch changed his mind after I explained my limitations. I don't blame him but I also refuse to feel sorry for myself anymore.

Celiac has had a huge social impact on my life, both before and after I figured out what was wrong with me. But as a wise man once said, we can let life's experiences make us better, or we can let them make us bitter. There was a while there where I let celiac make me bitter. Life wasn't fair and I felt cheated, but that was the wrong way to look at it. Now, I choose to let it make me a better person. I am thankful every day that my body has rebounded from the myopathy that destroyed my muscles and made every step painful. I am grateful that I rarely get sores in my mouth anymore, even when I am served contaminated food, which is rare. Many aspects of my social life may be limited, but I can now participate in all the physical activities that I had to give up before. I can run, I can rollerblade, I can play Get it Bitch style tennis. So I can't share a plate of fried appetizers and a pitcher of beer with friends, oh fucking well!

Chapter Twenty-Six

A Haunting Case

Many years ago, before I discovered that I am not cut out to work nine to five in a cubicle farm that sucked the soul right out of my body, I worked as a case manager for senior and disability services. Towards the end of my time there I had a client whose case still haunts me to this day. She was in her mid-twenties, with two young children. She had worked hard to go to school and become a dental hygienist. She bought a beautiful home and furnished it accordingly. And then, all of a sudden, her body was ravaged with pain. Her joints and muscles were in constant agony. She couldn't work anymore. Her mother had to come and care for her and her children because she was basically bedridden. Her doctor diagnosed her with Rheumatoid Arthritis and Fibromyalgia.

I remember thinking at the time that something wasn't right. But I was just a case manager, not a medical doctor so of course I didn't say anything. What could I say anyway? While I was struggling with lower back pain at the time I was still years away from experiencing many of the same symptoms she was suffering from.

Now, looking back, I can't help but wonder if her life could have been saved by eliminating gluten or some other offending food. What if she had had a friend like mine who had set her on the path to an elimination diet and healing? Of course, maybe she really did have R.A. and fibro. Maybe. But maybe she didn't. Or maybe she had R.A. because of undiagnosed celiac. Plenty of people with untreated celiac go on to develop other autoimmune diseases, and this is likely since they unknowingly continue to eat what basically amounts to a poison for their body.

This former client of mine is the first person I thought of when I discovered what was wrong with me. I could have ended up just like her. I was well on my way. Before I discovered the Paleo AIP diet, I could see disability in my future. I cut work back to the bare minimum number of hours that would still pay the bills, but even that was still more than the maximum my body could handle. I wondered how much longer I would be able to work before I would be forced to apply and fight for Social Security Disability. I worried that my children would suffer more than they already were. Who would take care of them if, like her, I was bedridden from pain? Now I wonder, would she have been able to return to her normal life if someone had introduced her to the same diet? Would she have gotten her life back if her doctors had been trained to look for celiac? I can only hope that she has found healing somehow. I can only hope that this book will help other people out there who are suffering like I was, like I think she was, find the healing they need.

Chapter Twenty-Seven

Your Health, Your Hands

When a person has been sick a long time, there are those moments they look back on with hindsight and think, "I should have known something more serious was wrong." I have more moments like this than I can count.

One of the first was when I was a junior in high school. I had some friends over for a sleepover and they wanted to go down to the pool after a small meal. But the last thing I wanted to do was wear a swimsuit after eating. You see, every time I ate my belly would distend. So much so that, as a thin girl with a normally flat tummy, I looked like I was months pregnant even back in high school. I thought this was normal. It was just the bulk of food jutting out right? Didn't this happen to everyone? My friends looked at me like I was crazy when I mentioned why I would rather wait. But I wasn't crazy, it wasn't my imagination, and it wasn't normal at all. I didn't know it at the time, but the reason my belly swelled up during digestion was because of the damage that had been done to my intestines. Whereas I thought this was normal because I had experienced it for so long, none of my friends knew what I was talking about because their guts were normal and undamaged. Their tummies did not pouch out after they ate. They did not look pregnant in their swimsuits.

After I found out was wrong with me I looked back on times like that one and beat myself up for not recognizing sooner that there was something serious wrong with my health. If I had, maybe I would have gotten a diagnosis sooner. Maybe I wouldn't have suffered as much.

I can't change the past. No one can. I must let it go. Yes, I wish I could have enjoyed my life more without the years of pain and illness. Yes, my kids' childhoods would have been richer had I been able to live a full life back then. But dwelling on that won't get me anywhere. All I can do is move forward and be grateful for the miracle of health that I have now.

That and share the miracle, so that others may find healing.

Maybe you are one of those people, maybe someone close to you is. True, I am making quite the assumption right now. But why else would you be reading this unless you suspect food intolerances and/or an autoimmune disease are at play in your life?

Don't accept a diagnosis that you know isn't right. If I had accepted my doctor's explanation for the sores in my mouth they would never have gone away. This would have reinforced the misdiagnosis because herpes never goes away. How many different pills and rinses would my doctor have sent me to the pharmacy for had I just gone along with it? Would she have ever realized that her diagnosis was wrong? Or would she just have told me that I was one of the unlucky few whose symptoms would not lessen with treatment?

And if I had agreed to take blood pressure medication, what kind of damage could have been done to my body by ingesting unnecessary medication? What would my liver and kidney function be like if I had become dependent on NSAIDs for the arthritis she claimed I had? Or if I had continued to take the muscle relaxers and anti-inflammatories she prescribed for my back?

How many more prescriptions would she have written if she had taken the time to listen to my symptoms instead of rushing me out the door? Would she have decided the scabs on my scalp were psoriasis and put me on Humira? What kind of rinse or pill could she have thought up for my dry mouth? In a way, I am grateful that she did not take the time to listen. If she had, she may have diagnosed me with the wrong life-altering auto-immune disease and I would have believed her and would never have discovered the elimination diet or the fact that what ails me comes from gluten ingestion. I would have just kept getting worse and worse. Not to mention the pills and specialists that would have been involved.

It makes me wonder, how many people are languishing on disability, popping pill after pill to treat symptoms, when relief from their disease is as simple as eliminating a food? How many people are suffering without a diagnosis because their doctors refuse to listen? Are you one of them? Is someone you love?

If the symptoms in the next chapter sound all too familiar, I highly recommend an elimination diet focused on healing leaky gut. At the very least, get rid of gluten, soy, and dairy for 30 days and see how you feel. Put them back one at a time. Follow the instructions for the oral challenge. I did it wrong and got terribly sick. Don't do the oral challenge the way I did. Be careful. Know that reactions can get worse over time. The point is to get better, not worse.

It is your health, and it is in your hands. The ultimate responsibility for your wellbeing is yours and yours alone. It may be your doctor's job to diagnose and treat you, but that doesn't mean they will. This is especially true for those with celiac disease.

Statistics say we are only one percent of the population but the disease is largely ignored in medical school and most doctors are not trained to recognize it. According to celiac.org, 80% of people with celiac in the U.S. are undiagnosed.

I should have been diagnosed as a teenager when I presented with chronic stomach pains and diarrhea. Celiac should be considered for anyone with those symptoms. It should be ruled out before a patient is sent home with a diagnosis of stress, which is really just a catch-all for when a doctor either doesn't know how or doesn't care to uncover the real problem. There was a twenty-year delay between the first time I went to the doctor for symptoms of celiac and when I finally got relief. It would have been longer had I relied on my doctor (if ever). The average celiac goes ten years before they receive a proper diagnosis. Some people go their entire lives and never know. Some people die from complications of the disease because they were never diagnosed.

Don't become a statistic. If something isn't right and your doctor isn't helping, take control of your health today!

Chapter Twenty-Eight

A Random Array of Symptoms

This is the list of random, seemingly unconnected symptoms that I gave my friend to share with her colleagues. Some of them are embarrassing. Others are weird. There is no rhyme or reason to the order of the list and I have not edited it but I have made some notes in regular font. This is exactly what I sent her and what she shared with her peers:

35 y/o female, 5'3" currently 127 lbs. Two live births, one miscarriage. (They always ask this so I figured it could be relevant.)

Current medications/vitamins: RSO (Rick Simpson Oil) 2xs/day as of 03/17, Powder AIP friendly Calcium, Vitamin C, and Magnesium, Vitamin D drops as of beginning AIP elimination diet, prior to that I was taking regular pill form of these along with a multivitamin.

Diet Changes: Began shifting towards a Paleo Auto Immune Protocol elimination diet a few weeks ago. (No grains, soy, nuts, seeds, dairy, nightshades, etc.) One week ago, slipped and had a Ultimate Cheeseburger from Jack in the Box and ulcers started to develop the next day after having cleared up. Not sure if this is connected but worth noting.

Between diet changes and RSO I have noticed a drastic change. Such as the last flare of ulcers in my mouth was not as intense as previous ones and seems to have cleared up without a second round of sores (there are usually at least two or three waves of sores.) Also, every step I take doesn't hurt and I am not waking up in the middle of the night with burning elbows. Though I imagine if I stop taking the RSO the pain will return. (RSO was a godsend at the time. It's anti-inflammatory properties helped me deal with the pain both before I went on the AIP diet as well as during it. I stopped taking it a couple of months later, after I knew I wasn't dealing with R.A. or lupus or any of the other auto-immune disorders. By then my body had healed enough that I didn't really need the pain relief anymore.)

Symptoms:

Mouth ulcers- Began January or February 2015 and have come in multiple flares since then (sores in my mouth more often than not during 2015). A wave of 20 to 30 small sores will form or sometimes some as big as a dime will form under my tongue or next to my gums and when that wave starts to heal another will come so that I have had a mouth full of sores for over a month causing nutritional deficiencies and weight loss. (I was 148 before the sores took their toll and I could barely eat.) Under my tongue scabs will form over ulcers on the frenulum. Texture of my mouth and tongue changes during outbreaks, becoming rough. Tongue especially becomes tender, cracked, and dry. Only h/x of canker sores is when eating tons of citrus fruits especially pineapple. No h/x of cold sores. At last visit, provider said they are a type of herpes that flare up with stress. I asked for blood test, results not back yet. Regardless would not explain the rest of my symptoms and I take issue with stress being a trigger because they have not been happening when I am actually under stress. There have been plenty of stressful times in my life but this past year has not been a stressful one. In the past, I have also gotten small single ulcers in my nose which doc said was from allergies.

Ulcers began after taking Meloxicam and Baclofen for back/hip pain. At the time, I thought they were caused by the Meloxicam so I stopped taking it but they came back anyway.

Enamel loss- I have always had healthy strong teeth, no issue with cavities. March of last year I noticed four cavities from acid erosion (not infected). I have since lost an enormous amount of enamel on all of my teeth, especially along the gumline, despite paying more attention to oral care.

Skin writer's disease/dermatographic urticaria- Noticed in Feb/March 2015. It's not active all of the time but when it is I can write words in my skin with a piece of plastic or my fingernail and in ten minutes or so they will welt up so that you can read it and it will usually be red and itchy. I will also get itchy welts in the pattern of whatever is irritating my skin.

Burning pain in elbows- three to nine months. R elbow began hurting while working in a brewery, from hammering bungs, although brewer said it shouldn't cause it to hurt and no one else had this issue. L elbow started hurting about three months ago (hammering bungs only done with R arm). Now I'm waking up in the middle of the night with elbows in burning pain. (No longer waking up from pain and pain has decreased substantially since starting RSO. Ibuprofen and naproxen did not help much.) (At the time, I didn't know that it was gluten that was causing the elbow to burn so I gave RSO all of the credit for relieving the inflammation in my joints.)

Random skin stuff- Occasional hives. Body acne. Always have little bumps/pustules around my knees, arms, etc. Currently have a strange bump on the outer part of my L outer labia- just on the skin, not on mucous *membranes. It doesn't hurt or itch or pop like a pimple it's just there. It had a twin on the R outer labia but it came off and it was just skin.*

Dull headache- *Not sure how long I've had it, seems like on and off for a couple of months or so.*

Back/hip/butt/leg pain- *Began with minor back pain in 2010. Consistently worsened so that hips constantly hurt, nearly every step hurts, muscle cramping so intense you can feel the knots in my lower back, hips, and buttocks on the right side. Left side occ hurts but doesn't really compare. Hurts especially bad after work (bartender, on feet all the time, though total intensity of pain increased after working a desk job...). Exercise helps but the threshold appears to be hours a day of exercise and stretching and this still doesn't fix the problem, just makes it less horrible. At its worst I am in so much pain after a shift that I can't even sit on the couch. I was taking Epsom salt baths every night just to stop the tears. Pain radiates from my hips through my lower back and butt and down my R leg. R leg will also go numb while standing—standing still extremely painful but so is sitting and walking. However, in spite of this ridiculous muscle cramping I am very flexible for my age.*

This has improved greatly since taking RSO (and going on the diet). I also took RSO for a few months in the spring of 2015 (this was also when I was on the remineralization diet) *and noticed the same dramatic relief and was able to exercise and get back to normal weight of 130 (I was overweight at 145 in Jan 2015 due to extreme back pain barely able to move after work, weight has never been an issue for me prior). When I stopped taking the RSO* (and went off the remineralization diet) *that time the pain slowly came back so that I was in just as much pain Jan 2016 as Jan 2015.* (At the time that I wrote out these symptoms I had not made the connection between the limited carb diet I was also on at the time.)

Aside from Meloxicam and Baclofen (which seemed to make it worse) I was also given Vicodin (it made me way too fucking happy!) *It didn't really help and changed my personality so I didn't continue that medication either. I have tried a variety of NSAIDS with very little effectiveness.*

Overall, before starting the RSO and diet change I felt like I was 60 or 70 years old (this was a grave underestimate—only now that I am healed do I realize just how much pain I was in—90 is much more reasonable), *just in constant pain and tired from the pain waking me up. Getting out of bed in the morning I was very stiff and had to get up slow like an elderly woman.*

Pain behind knee- I went for a really long walk 02/13 (of 2015). It shouldn't still be sore and weak.

Dandruff/scabs on scalp- On and off past year. Seems to coincide with flares in mouth ulcers. I have never had an issue with dandruff previously.

Hands- stiff joints/weak hands/lack of dexterity- past year or so. I have been bartending and working in food service for a long time though.

Fatigue- Exhausted all of the time. If I work during the day I don't have energy to do anything after. If I work at night I sleep the whole next day. Sleeping ten to twelve hours a night when I can. (This has improved since starting RSO and sleep quality has improved.)

Hearing- Periods where I feel like I'm under water or words just sound mumbled. I have not been checked for wax buildup or regular hearing loss.

Stomach issues- ongoing stomach issues since I was a teenager- nausea, cramping, abdominal pain, diarrhea, told most likely stress when I went in at 16. I was under a lot of stress at home at the time but I continued to have issues with stomach/digestion whether I was under stress or not. I have also had issues with appetite, being unable to eat, especially when super hungry, and there have been times when I am so hungry and trying to eat but no appetite and feeling like gagging while trying to choke food down. 2010 or 2011 I had an acute issue for a few months where it felt like my food wasn't digesting. My stomach was swelling up. I was puking a lot and it was thick, not as processed as puke usually is. Also constipation alternating with diarrhea. Blood tests and ultrasound- nothing. Doc said probably stress again. Job was super stressful but even at times when I am not under stress I have had issue with my stomach swelling up, extreme bloating (not menstruation related) and it feels like my food isn't digesting and I will have constipation alternating with diarrhea. This happens once to three times a year and doesn't seem to coincide with stress.

Eyes- pingueculas on both eyes (allergies? Contacts?) H/x of extremely dry eyes. I had to stop wearing contacts for a few years because my eyes were too dry. Currently can't wear them very long. Eye Dr. said I had inflammation that closed off the oil glands in my eyelids. Rx for eyedrops two or three times, don't recall what they were though.

Blood pressure- consistently 120/80 until Jan 2015. I was in a lot of pain at the time and it was pretty high but I don't recall how high. Going to the MD has always stressed me out but lately I've been really anxious about it, my heart starts racing when I just call to make an appointment. A lot of this is *fear that I am not going to be heard and will end up disabled from lack of diagnosis/treatment but also just a general anxiety about doctors as people who can inform me that I am going to die or have some terrible disease. Because of this I am unable to get an accurate BP reading as I start freaking out just seeing the machine. I was feeling like my heart was pounding a lot in general as well so I went off hormonal birth control and cut out coffee but as of my last appointment a week ago it was super high (169 over something) don't know how much of this is anxiety vs. actual hypertension.*

As you can see, I was a hot mess. There were times I didn't think I would ever feel normal again. And without my help from my friend and the elimination diet, there's a good chance I wouldn't have. There is a good chance I would have ended up disabled.

No more beer, no more doughnuts, no more cake, no more flour tortillas or burritos or chile rellenos . . . it's a long list of things I loved and can no longer put in my body, but it is worth it. Almost every single symptom on this list has cleared up since I kicked gluten out of my life. My blood pressure is normal. I do not have arthritis. My back pain is gone. The scabs on my scalp are gone. The sores in my mouth are gone. They used to return any time I experience accidental ingestion (if I got glutened, in other words). But the longer it has been since I went gluten free, the less I see them. Now if I get glutened the first symptoms I experience are bloating, nausea, and diarrhea. Joint and back pain usually follow within a day or two. But other than that, my stomach has healed tremendously and I have normal bowel movements now. If you've ever been plagued with stomach issues, you know what a blessing that is.

And I have ankles! I didn't even know I had regular ankles underneath the edema that celiac caused. Before going off gluten my ankles had two states: swollen & extra swollen. I was a skinny girl with cankles for as long as I can remember. Now instead of a dimple on the inside of each, I can see the bone that normal people have.

There are no more weird bumps on my knees or arms and body pimples have all but disappeared. I can hear again. It no longer sounds like I am always under water. No more dry eyes either—instead of what felt like sandpaper in my eyes, I have normal, natural lubrication.

I still experience skin writer's disease but if that's the worst symptom to stick around then I truly have nothing to complain about. While skin writer's is an autoimmune reaction, it is harmless and can actually be kind of cool. I mean, I can write words in my skin with a cocktail straw. Not many people can do that. My clothes do leave welts on my skin, especially socks and bras and the seams on tight pants, but that is such a miniscule thing compared to where I was a year and a half ago!

The list of possible symptoms with untreated celiac seems to be never ending. While I had plenty of them, I did not have them all, by far. Estimates of possible symptoms with celiac range from two to three hundred seemingly random and disconnected symptoms. Because of the specific way that celiac does its damage, it affects everyone differently. An exhaustive list may never be possible since some symptoms are experienced by so few people that they are not yet recognized as possible celiac reactions, but I have attempted to collect the most common possible symptoms here:

Digestive symptoms:
- abdominal distention
- abdominal pain
- acid reflux and heartburn
- bloating
- chronic diarrhea
- constipation
- gas
- nausea
- stools which are light in color, fatty, and smell awful, or float
- vomiting
- weight loss or gain/unstable weight

Non-digestive symptoms:

- ADHD
- alopecia (hair loss)
- anemia/iron deficiency
- anxiety
- arthritis/joint pain
- ataxia (trouble with muscle coordination)
- balance problems from injury to the nervous system

- bone pain, osteomalacia (softening of bone tissue), osteoporosis (loss of bone density)
- brain fog
- canker sores/oral ulcers
- certain cancers including intestinal and lymphoma
- cognitive impairment from injury to the nervous system
- depression
- dermatitis herpetiformis (itchy rash with blisters)
- developmental delay
- delayed puberty
- eczema
- enamel damage/defects/discoloration
- fatigue
- headaches or migraines
- hyposplenism
- infertility/miscarriage
- irritability
- lactose intolerance
- liver problems/biliary tract disorders
- missed periods/delayed puberty
- muscle pain/myopathy (including misdiagnosis of fibromyalgia)
- peripheral neuropathy (numbness, tingling, and/or in the hands and feet)
- seizures
- short stature
- vitamin deficiency from malabsorption (which is what causes the non-intestinal symptoms. For example, deficiencies in magnesium and other vitamins and minerals is responsible for the myopathy that ravaged the muscles in my back and legs.)

For a checklist that can be emailed to your doctor, visit
https://celiac.org/celiac-disease/resources/checklist/

Chapter Twenty-Nine

Hope for a Cure

Many years ago, back when I was still trying to force myself to fit into office life, I had a co-worker who was a whizz at finding the most off the wall, random, but super interesting articles, which he would proceed to share with the rest of us. One day he brought to our attention the personal narrative of someone who claimed to have cured his asthma with hookworms.

Yup. You read that right. Asthma. Cured by hookworms.

Mmmmkay.

The author ascribed to the theory that diseases like asthma are so much more prevalent in Western societies because we are too clean. He claimed that hookworms provide some sort of valuable service for humans that prevents asthma, among other modern diseases, thus making for a symbiotic relationship.

He went on a mission to get himself some hookworms.

I don't remember where he went, somewhere in some developing nation where incidence of hookworm infection is super high. But he didn't just immerse himself among the locals and pick it up naturally the way they did, from just living life at its most basic level.

Nope. He took off his shoes and walked bare foot through the trenches where people relieved themselves. There was no way he was leaving without some damn hookworms.

He returned home, back to the good old U.S. of A., full of all these hookworms. This was many years ago that I read this article, so please excuse my fuzzy memory of the details. I don't recall how he knew exactly that he had successfully become infested with the little worms, whether there was some sort of test he did of his fecal matter or just a visual inspection. I don't really want to remember that part anyway.

And he claimed it worked. He claimed that as long as he kept a healthy community of hookworms living in his belly he was asthma free.

Now why the hell did I share this story?

Take a guess . . . yup, in the throes of gluten cravings I thought back on that strange guy and his willingness to walk through fecal matter and I wondered if hookworms could be used to treat celiac too. One Google search later and I found a scientific article about . . . oh yeah, celiac put into regression by our good old pals the hookworms!

The article theorized that the presence of the worms in the intestines did something to interfere with the autoimmune response that targets the villi. (https://www.sciencedaily.com/releases/2014/09/140925100929.htm) (https://research.jcu.edu.au/bmdt/publications/publications-1/giacomin-australian-science-april-2015)

Now no, I am not about to go traipsing barefoot through any roadside ditches or open sewers. But who knows maybe I'll get lucky and pick some up while travelling. As I write this I am backpacking through Central America, careful to leave my shoes off as much as possible, in hopes of maybe catching a few little helper hookworms along the way. Can't hurt right? Okay, hookworms aren't harmless, but in my case the good they could do is worth overlooking the small chance of illness that they bring along.

Of course, the scientific article did not recommend hookworms as treatment for celiac.

Darn it!

Instead, the authors hoped that the subject would be studied further to develop some sort of treatment based on the body's positive reaction to the little worms.

Still, I'll take a few hookworms if it means I can drink beer and eat burritos and churros and French fries and grilled cheese sandwiches and that crispy greasy thin crust pizza that was so popular in the 80's. And a chocolate chip calzone. Definitely a chocolate chip calzone.

Hookworms are nothing compared to human sacrifice, right?

Meanwhile, if a medical cure is found, Hoorah! If not, well at least I have already had one miracle. I have my health back. I feel young again. That's all that matters.

What about a maintenance treatment that allows the patient to eat gluten without consequence as long as they take a pill every day? Daily medication is the route most often used in Western medicine, the most likely result of hookworm research would be such.

Side effects may include drowsiness, trouble breathing, irregular heartbeat, panic and anxiety attacks, thinning of hair in both men and women, depression, suicidal ideation, liver and/or kidney failure, catatonia, and anal leakage.

Ok I'm being facetious again. I don't know what the actual side effects would be. But they do always seem to be worse than whatever it is the medication is supposed to cure, right?

Time will tell if a cure will be developed. In the meantime, I am just glad that I can live a pain free, active life again!

Chapter Thirty

Conclusion

True, this is my story of self-diagnosis. To get an official diagnosis, I would need to have my lower intestine biopsied and my villi examined by a qualified expert (false negatives are common when doctors do not take enough samples). An accurate biopsy of my villi would require me to go on a gluten inclusive diet for months. Three to six servings a day of something that even in the smallest increments makes me extremely ill, for months? No thank you! If just a little contamination, a few secret dashes of soy sauce, are enough to leave me clutching my stomach why would I subject myself to such a thing? An official diagnosis is not worth months of ulcers in my mouth or the cloud of anger, confusion, and self-loathing that would wrap itself around my brain. It's not worth destroying my muscles with myopathy, my back aching with every step, or my joints burning. It isn't worth any more damage to my teeth or heart.

Six months after I discovered the root of my health problems, I met with my gynecologist for that annual exam that is so important. When I reported my symptoms, how they were relieved by a gluten-free diet, and how awful the consequences of even a small amount of gluten were, she agreed with my self-diagnosis and said that she would put celiac in my chart. I'm not sure how that works without a biopsy, but I know that neither my body or my psyche could tolerate one and she agreed.

How do I know that I am suffering from celiac and not just gluten intolerance without a biopsy? Well I don't know for sure in the clinical sense. But I know that the erosion of enamel from my teeth is a sure sign of malabsorption, which happens when celiac damages the villi to the point where they can no longer properly absorb vitamins and minerals. Furthermore, during the year it took to fully recover, I noticed a huge difference in how I felt when I forgot to take vitamins like magnesium and Vitamin D. I also noticed way better outcomes in sunny climates when I get my Vitamin D from the sun instead of a pill. Anecdotally, my symptoms were also quite extreme for an "intolerance". The level of pain in my body was above and beyond anything I've ever read or heard attributed to gluten intolerance. Of course, healing is more important than a technical diagnosis.

If you are experiencing digestive and/or autoimmune symptoms that your doctor is ignoring, you might have to take your health in your own hands like I did. Don't let a slew of misdiagnosis keep you sick. Is it worth worrying about a technical diagnosis when you could get better instead? If you are suffering like I was, an elimination diet might just save your life.

If others receive healing after reading about my experience then what I went through will be worth it. Celiac is a terrible disease to have, true, but it is manageable. I am so happy that I have learned to be grateful once again. It could be so much worse! Every day I am thankful that I do not have a medication routine or appointments with specialists. Although there was a long delay in my diagnosis, it still came before serious damage was done. Disability is no longer in my future. I have control over this disease, it does not control me!

Printed in Great Britain
by Amazon

86388563R00052